ASSISTED CONCEPTION

Assisted Conception

Research, ethics and law

Edited by
JENNIFER GUNNING
Cardiff Law School

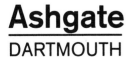

DARTMOUTH

Aldershot • Burlington USA • Singapore • Sydney

Published by
Dartmouth Publishing Company Limited
Ashgate Publishing Ltd
Gower House
Croft Road
Aldershot
Hants GU11 3HR
England

Ashgate Publishing Company
131 Main Street
Burlington, VT 05401-5600 USA

Ashgate website: http://www.ashgate.com

British Library Cataloguing in Publication Data
Assisted conception : research, ethics and law
　　1.Human reproductive technology - European Union countries
　　2.Human reproductive technology - Research - Law and
　　legislation - European Union countries 3.Human reproductive
　　technology - Research - Moral and ethical aspects -
　　European Union countries
　　I.Gunning, Jennifer
　　341.7'6757

Library of Congress Control Number: 00-134486

ISBN 0 7546 2149 9

Printed and bound by Athenaeum Press, Ltd.,
Gateshead, Tyne & Wear.

Contents

v

List of Tables

List of Contributors

Inez de Beaufort is Professor of Health Care Ethics at the Medical Faculty of the Erasmus University in Rotterdam. She is a member of the Dutch Health Council, the Dutch Council of Health Care and the Medical Ethics Committee of the Royal Dutch Medical Association and the Dutch Commission for Ethics and research.

Bruno Brambati is Head of the Prenatal Diagnosis Unit at the First Institute of Obstetrics and Gynecology, "L.Mangiagalli" Clinic, University of Milan, where his research has focused on the fetal diagnosis of genetic diseases. He is a member of the Board of the International Society for Prenatal Diagnosis and is a member of the Expert Group on Fetal Diagnosis of the WHO Hereditary Disease Program.

Wybo J. Dondorp studied theology and ethics. He works as an ethicist at the bureau of the Health Council of the Netherlands in The Hague. He is scientific secretary of the Standing Committee on Medical Ethics and Health Law, and of several of the Council's ad-hoc committees.

Veronica English is the Deputy Head of Medical Ethics at the British Medical Association. Her role is to provide ethical advice for doctors in response to inquiries and to prepare guidance and reports on a range of ethical issues. Before joining the BMA she worked for seven years in the regulation of infertility treatment with both the voluntary and statutory regulatory authorities.

Jennifer Gunning was for three years Secretary of the Voluntary Licensing Authority for Human in vitro Fertilisation and Embryology. Subsequently she wrote a report for the UK government on human IVF and embryo research and related issues to provide information for Parliament during the passage of the Human Fertilisation and Embryology Bill. She is now working as an independent consultant and is a research associate in medical law and ethics at Cardiff Law School.

Inga Hanschel is a trainee lawyer in Germany at the Freiburg State Court. Until the end of 1999 she was employed at the Max-Planck-Institute for Foreign and International Law in the Department of Law and Medicine.

Martin H. Johnson was for six years, until recently, a member of the Human Fertilisation and Embryology Authority of the UK, with direct experience of the regulatory process and the impact of ethical decision making on it. He has also undertaken licensed research using human embryos and gametes. He is Professor of Reproductive Sciences at the University of Cambridge.

Pascal Kamina is Assistant Professor (Maître de Conférences) at the University of Poitiers. where he teaches EC law and Intellectual Property related courses. His interest in the French "bioethics" laws of 1994 and in the regulation of assisted conception techniques comes primarily from his research in the fields of biotechnology and family law.

Sheila A.M. McLean is Director of the Institute of Law and Ethics in Medicine at the University of Glasgow.

Derek Morgan is Reader in Health Care Law & Jurisprudence at Cardiff Law School. He is a member of the British Medical Association's Medical Ethics Committee, and has chaired and contributed to a number of the Association's Working Parties since 1994. He was a member of the Chief Medical Officer's Expert Group on Cloning and was the founding convenor of the Society of Public Teachers of Law, Medical Law Group.

Maurizio Mori is Editor of Bioetica Rivista Interdisciplinare, Secretary of the Consulta di Bioetica, and is in charge of the "Bioetica" branch of the research center "Politeia" in Milan. He is visiting professor in the philosophy of law at the Law Faculty of Alessandria.

Linda Nielsen has recently stepped down after three years as chairman of the Danish Council of Ethics. She is a Professor in the Law Faculty of the University of Copenhagen. Her professional interests are in the areas of family and health law.

Judit Sándor is an Hungarian Medical Lawyer. She teaches graduate students from Central and Eastern European countries at the Central European University and teaches medical law, health care law, human rights, legal policy and medical ethics in different faculties in Budapest.

Her main research interests are patients' rights, medical negligence, reproductive rights, genetics, and anti-discrimination laws.

André Van Steirteghem has been, since 1983, Scientific Director of the Centre for Reproductive Medicine at the Medical Campus of the Dutch-speaking Brussels Free University (VUB).   He is full Professor in Embryology and Reproductive Biology at the Medical School and Director of the Research Unit on Reproductive Biology.

Guido de Wert is an Ethicist, and Senior Research Fellow at the Institute for Bioethics, University of Maastricht, The Netherlands.

Preface

Assisted conception is an area where it often seems that all the ethical and legal issues have been covered and then the technology advances once more, such as the advent of cloning, and the discussions start all over again. It seemed that the opening for signature of the European Convention on Human Rights and Biomedicine in April 1997 marked the end of an era, and it did in a way. In article 18 the use of human embryos was addressed and, for those countries signing and ratifying the Convention, the opportunities for future research restricted. But the consequences of this for infertility patients have not really been thought about.

Assisted reproduction technology is not static. Approaches to the problems of infertility are becoming ever more sophisticated, for instance using immature gametes or their progenitor cells. This technology must be proved safe before is transferred to routine clinical practice. Those countries restricting or prohibiting research on human embryos are less likely to have the research and training base required to ensure safety and competence in the initial application of these technologies in practice. There is therefore a risk that patients may become the unsuspecting subjects of experiment.

To test the plausibility of this hypothesis a group of partners from across Europe joined, with EC funds, to undertake a project looking at therapeutic research in assisted conception. Two workshops were held, the first looking at current issues and the second looking ahead to future avenues of research, their ethics and regulation. This book is an anthology of some of the papers presented during the course of the project.

The book has been divided into three parts addressing research, ethics and law with, at the beginning of each, an overview of issues that arose in discussion and which are addressed in the subsequent chapters. The aim has been to offer some new perspectives rather than to go over old ground.

It seems that there may be concern about clinical standards in those countries without a strong research and training base. Although this can, in part, be overcome through reproductive tourism where patients seek unavailable or a higher standard of treatment in clinics situated in countries other than their own. The increasingly free movement of goods and services across Europe will undoubtedly see the greater commodification of medical services with customers seeking treatment where it suits them best. However, this can only be done at some cost and is really only an opportunity, at present, for the comfortably off who can afford treatment in private clinics. A more reasonable alternative, and one which is to some extent already underway, is that practitioners should travel to the most advanced clinics to train in the latest techniques.

While it is clear that there will never be a consensus on the status of the human embryo nor on who should have access to the different forms of assisted conception treatment, as different countries have different cultural norms, there is a willingness to accept some form of technical standardization across Europe. This would appear to be an opportunity that should not be missed.

Acknowledgements

First of all I would like to acknowledge my partners in the TRAC project who made invaluable contributions to the running and success of the project and to this volume. They are, Bruno Brambati, Inez de Beaufort, Panagiota Dalla-Vorgia, Veronica English, Inga Hanschel and Andre Van Steirteghem. In particular, I would to thank Panagiota Dalla-Vorgia and her family for their helpfulness and hospitality and for the immaculate organisation of the TRAC workshop in Athens in April 1999.

I would also like to acknowledge the co-operation and contributions of the other contributors to this volume and the participants at the two TRAC workshops.

Thanks go, too, to Hugh Whittall, now back at the HFEA, for his help and encouragement when he was responsible for the TRAC project while at the European Commission.

The TRAC project was supported by EC Contract No. BMH4-CT98-3580.

List of Abbreviations

AH	Assisted hatching
AID	Artificial insemination by donor
AIH	Artificial insemination by husband
AMP	Assistance médicale à la procréation
ART	Assisted reproductive technology
CPH	Code de la santé publique
CVS	Chorionic villus sampling
ESC	Embryonic stem cells
EschG	Embryonenschutzgesetz
ESHRE	European Society for Human Reproduction and Embryology
FISH	Fluorescence in situ hybridization
GIFT	Gamete intra-fallopian transfer
HFE (Act)	Human Fertilisation and Embryology Act
HFEA	Human Fertilisation and Embryology Authority
HOS	Hypo-osmotic swelling
ICSI	Intra-cytoplasmic sperm injection
IVF-ET	In vitro fertilization and embryo transfer
IVM	In vitro maturation
KEMO	National Ethical Review Board (Netherlands)
MAP	Medically assisted procreation
MESA	Microsurgical sperm aspiration
MRC	Medical Research Council
mtDNA	Mitochondrial DNA
NABER	National Advisory Board on Ethics in Reproduction (USA)
PCR	Polymerase chain reaction
PGD	Preimplantation genetic diagnosis
PGS	Preimplantation genetic screening
PND	Prenatal diagnosis
PROST	Pro-nuclear stage transfer
RCOG	Royal College of Obstetricians and Gynaecologists
REC	Reproductive embryo cloning
SUZI	Subzonal insemination
TC	Therapeutic cloning
TESE	Testicular sperm extraction
TET	Tubal embryo transfer

THBR	Take home baby rate
TRAC	Therapeutic research in assisted conception
TUKEB	National Science and Research Ethics Council (Hungary)
VLA	Voluntary Licensing Authority
ZIFT	Zygote intra-fallopian transfer

INTRODUCTION

1 Introduction

JENNIFER GUNNING

Background

The European Convention on Human Rights and Biomedicine is a landmark in the regulation of assisted conception. It seeks to obtain a consensus, which will apply across its member states, and to have a far-reaching effect on medical practice across Europe. It was opened for signature in April 1997 and has now been signed by 28 member states and ratified by six. It came into force on 1 December 1999. Assisted conception services will be affected by Article 18, which specifically addresses research on embryos in vitro, stating that

1. Where the law allows research on embryos in vitro, it shall ensure adequate protection of the embryo.
2. The creation of human embryos for research purposes is prohibited.

Countries already having law in force, permitting the creation of embryos for research, before signing the Convention will be able to have a reservation on this article.

However, the implication is that the Convention would allow therapeutic research (see below for the definition used here) and research on spare embryos but forbid fundamental research, which may be essential to the safe development of new techniques. The development of new in vitro techniques involving the manipulation of gametes, for instance, would then be encouraged directly in the clinical context, as therapeutic research, without any knowledge as to their safety or efficacy except in countries where research is allowed.

Non-therapeutic research on the human embryo, in those countries where it is allowed, is subject to rigorous ethical and scientific scrutiny. In the United Kingdom, the Human Fertilisation and Embryology Act (1990) forbids the return to the uterus of any embryo which has been the subject of research. This is because, by definition, the results of research cannot be predicted and therefore may not be beneficial. Research involving the creation of human embryos is needed particularly in the development of

3

techniques involving gamete manipulation, such as ICSI with immature sperm, in order to determine that normal fertilization and embryonic development is likely to result. Allowing research on spare embryos, which have already been created for treatment purposes, is not appropriate for this type of research, which nevertheless underpins the safety of assisted conception techniques. This means that new techniques will have to be developed in the course of treatment.

Although therapeutic research is intended to be for the benefit of the individual in question, in fact, whether it is of real benefit to the individual is unknown. Often such procedures will be undertaken in the context of clinical treatment so that they are not subject to the same level of ethical and scientific scrutiny accorded to non-therapeutic research. In addition, the couple seeking assisted conception may, unknowingly, become part of the experiment. Article 1 of the Convention on Human Rights and Biomedicine states, as its purpose and object, that

> Parties to this convention shall protect the dignity and identity of all human beings, and guarantee everyone, without discrimination, respect for their integrity and other rights and fundamental freedoms with regard to the application of biology and medicine.

Therapeutic embryo research may have unexpected and unwanted long term effects which would affect the health or reproductive capacity of the resultant offspring. There is a possibility that, under the guise of therapeutic research, risks may be undertaken with embryos, which are implanted as part of treatment, because the fundamental research, which might have avoided that risk, is forbidden.

The TRAC project

Bearing in mind the above, we embarked upon a project to endeavor to ascertain whether there might be risks of infertility patients being exposed to insufficiently tested procedures and whether there really was still a need for fundamental research in this area; what legislative safeguards existed and whether European standards for treatment needed to be set. The project brought together clinicians, embryologists, lawyers and ethicists and their first task was to agree a definition of therapeutic research and other types of research, which would provide the background to discussion at two workshops. The definitions agreed were as follows.

In the development of new techniques for clinical practice there are at least three stages:

1. research is conducted on animals or on tissue or human material outside the body;
2. the procedure is used in clinical practice for the first time; and
3. the procedure becomes routine clinical practice.

With embryo research, the first stage includes carrying out new procedures on embryos in vitro and assessing the impact on their development with no intention of replacing them in the uterus. The second stage includes the first few cases where the embryos, having been subjected to the new procedure, are replaced in the uterus; this second stage is therapeutic research and was the subject of this research project.

As an example one may consider the development of intra-cytoplasmic sperm injection (ICSI). The first stage involved injecting oocytes in vitro, assessing their development, with no intention of replacing them. Once sufficient reassurance was obtained about safety and efficacy, a small number of procedures were carried out and the embryos replaced into the uterus for gestation. These cases were carefully monitored to provide further information in order to assess the technique before it reached the third stage of routine clinical practice.

The concern arising out of the Convention on Human Rights and Biomedicine is that stage 2 will be implemented too early because certain aspects of stage 1 will be prohibited in some countries.

Therapeutic research

Research which is intended to benefit the participant or subject.

Experimental therapy

It has been usual in the field of reproductive medicine for doctors to learn new techniques, such as laparoscopy or fetal sampling, by practicing on animals or, with their consent, on pregnant women undergoing an abortion. It is not clear that there is a parallel in assisted conception, particularly in those clinics which operate outside the academic environment. Patients treated early on in the phase of technology transfer are likely to become the subjects of experimental therapy with a lower chance of a successful outcome.

Non-therapeutic research

Generally non-therapeutic research is research which is not intended to benefit the individual. This takes two forms. In the context of this project it refers to the first stage of the process described above whereby the procedure is undertaken on oocytes or embryos in vitro with no intention to replace them in the uterus. In other types of research it may involve human subjects but with no benefit to the particular participant e.g. using healthy volunteers for research into conditions such as the common cold or for drug trials.

Applied research

Applied research is research with a particular clinical aim such as, with embryo research, improving the culture medium, developing techniques for preimplantation diagnosis, or developing new forms of treatment such as ICSI.

Pure research

Pure research is aimed at gaining a greater understanding of basic biological processes with no particular clinical aim. The knowledge arising from this type of basic research will, however, be used for designing applied research as described above.

Conclusions

The TRAC project aimed throughout to look at the question of therapeutic research in assisted conception from three perspectives; those of research, ethics and law. This book provides a selection of contributions to the project from these three perspectives.

Two workshops were held where the emphasis was on discussion but where presentations were given to provide the stimulus for discussion. A picture was obtained of the current state of ART provision in a number of countries across Europe and of typical success rates and current and possible future avenues of research involving human embryos were discussed. The status of the human embryo was not a principal focus of the ethical discussions, since this has already had widespread discussion, although it inevitably arose. Rather, the project focused more on the more practical aspects of ethics in the context of ART. Finally, comparisons were made between the different ways in which countries across Europe had, or had not, legislated on human embryo research and different approaches to and models of regulation considered.

It is clear that the provision of and access to assisted conception services varies from country to country. In some countries, such as the UK, provision is predominantly in the private sector with patients paying considerable sums for treatment. In others, such as Denmark, treatment is readily available with public funding although private clinics do exist. The success rate of treatment is also variable even in those countries with a good research base. Better understanding of embryo handling and culture is still needed. But the development of ART has not yet come to a standstill and the future direction of assisted conception will be dependent on research. New directions of research raise new ethical questions and, in the light of the European Convention on Human Rights and Biomedicine which will impose a more restrictive approach to research, regulation, particularly of the transfer of new technology into clinical practice, will become an important issue. But human embryo research and embryonic stem cell technology have the potential to benefit other areas of medicine than that of reproduction and it is evident that proper consideration needs to be given to the costs and benefits of such research and the ethical issues surrounding it before blanket prohibitions are put in place as a reaction to innovations which are not fully understood and often misrepresented by the media.

Relatively few European countries have introduced legislation addressing human embryo research, and even fewer have established regulatory bodies to oversee the clinical provision of ART, but 28 have signed the European Convention on Human Rights and Biomedicine. This might suggest that once, the status of the embryo has been recognized and human embryo research duly limited, other ethical issues related to assisted conception and its provision are in danger of being ignored. But the Convention also insists that patients should be assured the highest standards of treatment and that interventions should only be carried out in the light of free and informed consent.

At the end of the project a survey was carried out among those involved in the provision of assisted conception services and this revealed that there was consensus that some technical standardization across Europe was needed. The results of this survey are given in Chapter 18. Because of restrictive legislation in some countries not all assisted reproduction technologies are available to their patients. Some will inevitably travel to other countries, therefore, to seek treatment and they should have access to similar standards of facility, treatment and care, with similar chances of success, wherever they go. It is equally important that those who cannot afford the costs of reproductive tourism should at least have access to the best practice available. Some form of European standardization would help to achieve this.

Part I
RESEARCH

2 Overview: Human Embryo Research

BRUNO BRAMBATI AND ANDRE VAN STEIRTEGHEM

Regulation of embryo research and its transfer into clinical practice

In Europe different attitudes prevail regarding the regulation of human embryo research and the transfer of these research results into clinical practice. The attitudes in the United Kingdom, Belgium and Germany will be reviewed.

United Kingdom

In the UK research on human gametes and embryos used in studies on the process of fertilisation is regulated by the Human Fertilisation and Embryology (HFE) Act of 1990. The Act functions through a system of licensing for storage, for treatment or for research. There are relatively few prohibitions and the approach to legislation is fundamentally flexible. There are two underlying assumptions: (1) licensing is entrusted by Parliament (the lawmakers) to a non-elected body of people (The Human Fertilisation and Embryology Authority – HFEA) acting on Parliament's behalf. HFEA members have to accept the law administered by HFEA. (2) a legally pragmatic or ethically consequentialist view on complex issues with advantages and disadvantages discounts the possibility that specific prohibitions are often not in society's long term interest. HFEA's approach to legislation is very flexible and may interpret the law in relation to the current situation and may take into account continuous scientific advances. A new therapeutic technique, which involves the creation of embryos, cannot be used unless an application for a licence has been approved. This allows the HFEA to control the introduction and dissemination of new techniques fairly robustly. The application for a licence for a new technique must meet a general set of requirements; it is unlikely that centres would be granted licences for new techniques until they have demonstrated competence at standard techniques. The requirements include evidence

11

from work on animals, from research on human gametes and embryos (without replacement into patients)

- that the local operatives at the therapeutic centre have the skills required to carry out the technique efficiently
- that the patient population for the initial treatments must be specified
- that the patient information must be submitted together with details of how it will be used and
- that the consent form must be submitted.

If a technique is used without either enquiry or license application and the HFEA considers the technique to be new, the center is considered in breach of its license or, less likely, to have performed a licensable technique illegally. Thus, the HFEA can control the introduction and dissemination of new techniques fairly robustly.

Quality control is also applied on the well established techniques: clinical standards are monitored by a centralised data bank receiving data in real time from each clinical centre; a periodical audit is regularly organised.

Germany

The Embryo Protection Law (December 1990) includes a number of restrictions for clinical practice; this includes prohibition of egg donation, surrogacy and the fertilisation of an oocyte for any other purpose than the establishment of pregnancy. From the moment of the fusion of the two pronuclei the fertilised oocyte is considered as a human individual. The question whether research could be carried out before syngamy (the fusion of the two pronuclei), is irrelevant since experimentation is only possible on such fertilised oocytes if the procedure is undertaken for the well-being of the embryo itself, which would have to be replaced. The limited research possible in Germany involves certain aspects of in-vitro maturation of immature oocytes.

Belgium

A law on the protection of the human embryo in-vitro is still pending. Notwithstanding the current absence of legal framework, ethical recommendations for research on human embryos were already formulated in the mid-eighties: the Ethical Committee of the Belgian Fund for Medical Research adopted the recommendations of the British Warnock Committee.

Research projects on human gametes and embryos need prior approval of the local ethical committee. Several new procedures related to Assisted Reproductive Technology (ART) such as Intra-Cytoplasmic Sperm Injection (ICSI) and preimplantation genetic diagnosis (PGD) were correctly introduced into the clinic by self-regulation and continuous audit of the clinical and research activities. Clinical subzonal insemination (SUZI) was preceded by experimental assessment in the mouse. For ICSI, animal models were inappropriate and pre-clinical observations on ICSI embryos were carried out. The first clinical success with ICSI occurred in Belgium. Initially ICSI was carried out under strict conditions including prenatal diagnosis and a prospective follow-up of all the pregnancies and the children born. This ongoing study has allowed providing correct information of the outcomes of ICSI to prospective parents.

PGD, another novel procedure of the nineties, was developed into clinical practice after extensive pre-clinical evaluation and assessment of the different steps in the PGD procedure: embryo biopsy, single-cell genetic diagnosis using fluorescent in situ hybridization (FISH) or polymerase chain reaction (PCR). Like ICSI, clinical PGD should also be monitored very closely including the follow-up of the children born.

A proposal of law on the protection of human embryos in vitro was introduced in Parliament after approval by the Council of Ministers. It describes the framework in which research on supernumerary or in vitro created embryos can be carried out; research topics, which are possible or not possible, are also enumerated in the proposal of law. The flow chart for allowing research on human embryos includes approval by the Local Ethical Committee and evaluation by a Federal Commission.

Future directions in human embryo research

Three future areas involving research on human embryos will be discussed: pre-implantation genetic diagnosis, the case of the embryo in relation to the ethics of cloning and other future possible directions of human embryo research.

Preimplantation genetic diagnosis (PGD).

Since its introduction 10 years ago the number of centres offering PGD has grown steadily but slowly. So far there has been a lack of systematic longitudinal registration of the PGD activity world-wide. The absence of such data collection precludes an evaluation of the current status of PGD, which should still be considered as an experimental procedure. PGD aims towards the transfer of unaffected embryos. It would avoid the selective termination of pregnancies after prenatal diagnosis (by chorionic villus sampling or amniocentesis) in couples at high risk of transferring genetic diseases to their offspring. PGD, involving ART, is not without potential problems, such as risks related to IVF-ICSI and the embryo biopsy procedure, which is needed to obtain the diagnostic specimen. The success of PGD including its efficiency and accuracy is largely unknown. A systematic study of PGD has been initiated by the PGD consortium of the European Society of Human Reproduction and Embryology (ESHRE). The aims of the ESHRE consortium are described in chapter 3. A first report of the ESHRE PGD Consortium was published in December 1999 in the Journal of Human Reproduction.[1]

There are many possible future developments related to PGD including aneuploidy screening in human pre-implantation embryos, removal of blastomeres or trophoblast biopsy, uterine flushing of embryos, karyotyping of single cells, multiplex PCR to look simultaneously at different diseases, sex determination in embryos for non-medical indications, whole genome amplification, carrier selection in X-linked diseases, Y-chromosome deletions, mitochondrial DNA and gene therapy.

The case of the embryo in relation to the ethics of cloning

A wide variety of activities have been included under the general heading of 'cloning'. Those that involve the creation and use of embryos can be divided into two distinct types based on the ultimate objective. Where the objective is deliberately to create genetically identical individuals, this is often referred to as 'reproductive cloning'. This technique may, theoretically, be used either to create an individual with the same genetic make-up as an existing individual- by cell nuclear replacement techniques - or to deliberately produce monozygotic twins - either by cell nuclear replacement or embryo splitting - with the primary intention of increasing the number of embryos available for transfer in an IVF cycle. Although the ethical arguments differ, both of these techniques have been prohibited in a broad statement in the Additional Protocol to the Human Rights and Biomedicine Convention.

The second category of activities does not involve the creation of genetically identical individuals, but aims to produce an unlimited source of tissue for transplantation. It is proposed that undifferentiated embryonic stem cells, from early embryos, could be stimulated to differentiate into whatever type of tissue was needed - neural tissue for the treatment of degenerative diseases such as Parkinson's disease, bone marrow for leukaemia sufferers, islet cells for diabetes, muscle tissue for the repair of a damaged heart or skin for treating burns victims. A further development would be to produce tissue which was immunologically compatible to the recipient. This could be achieved by transferring the nucleus from one of the patient's own somatic cells into an enucleated donor egg which would then be stimulated to begin cell-division but only to the stage needed to separate and culture the embryonic stem cells. This would succeed, not only in overcoming the shortage of tissue for transplantation but also, because the cells would be generated using the patient's own DNA, the tissue would be fully compatible so there would be no need for the use of immunosuppressive drugs. This use of cloning techniques has potentially huge implications for a vast number of people.

Other future directions in human embryo research

Without considering their deeper ethical or legal implications possible new developments in human embryo research may include:

- Non-invasive methods for more efficient selection of spermatozoa, eggs or embryos which have the greatest potential for development. Criteria assessed have included tests for selection of immotile sperm, blood flow in the growing follicle, free radical production in fertilisation medium, location and size of pronuclei, blastomere morphology and division rate, metabolic activity, blastocyst formation in-vitro as well as the use of vital dyes.

- Improvement of embryo quality by improving the quality of culture media.

- Research to actively improve the quality of the embryo. This more controversial approach includes cytoplasmic or gene therapy.

- Research into the production of more embryos which may be achieved by in-vitro maturation of oocytes, the use of cadavers and fetuses as a source of oocytes, the use of embryonic stem cells as a source of gametes, maturation of human gametes in living incubators, the induction of cells to undergo meiosis in vitro, oocyte cryopreservation and embryo splitting.

- New technical routes to parenthood to satisfy new patterns of parenting.

- Improvement of implantation by procedures on the zona pellucida or the embryo itself.

- Advances in contraceptive technology would benefit all human beings. Many of the problems in the world stem from inexorably rising birth rates and in the difficulty of providing acceptable methods for safe, efficient, and reversible contraception.

These issues are considered in more detail in chapter 4.

Note

1   ESHRE PGD Consortium Steering Committee (1999) 'ESHRE Preimplantation Genetic Diagnosis (PGD) Consortium: preliminary assessment of data from January 1997 to September 1998', *Human Reproduction*, vol. 14, pp. 3138-3148.

3 Preimplantation Genetic Diagnosis

JENNIFER GUNNING

Introduction

The vast majority of pregnancies, whether conceived as a result of assisted conception or through normal sexual intercourse, proceeds without difficulty and results in the birth of a normal child. To help ensure the best outcome for their pregnancy, women may be offered a number of tests to check that their fetus is normal and healthy.

These prenatal tests generally fall into two categories; screening tests and diagnostic tests. Screening tests are carried out on the whole population or on a particular population which has a higher risk of transmitting a genetic disorder. Diagnostic tests are used to confirm pregnancy or to determine whether the fetus has a genetic disorder. Most testing will help women to decide whether to terminate a pregnancy if they are carrying an affected fetus or, if they wish to continue the pregnancy, attempt treatment if appropriate and enable doctors to decide how to treat the child when it is born.

Screening tests

Prenatal screening tests give information about the level of risk of the condition being screened for. Diagnostic tests may then be used to confirm or refute a positive result. The most commonly used screening tests are biochemical tests on maternal blood to determine the level of risk of Down's syndrome or neural tube defects and ultrasound scans which can pick up anomalies of fetal development which are indicative of chromosomal defects. Biochemical testing is usually undertaken at about 10-14 weeks of pregnancy and ultrasound screening at about 18 weeks. A positive result from these screening tests would then have to be confirmed using a more accurate diagnostic test such as amniocentesis.

Diagnostic tests

Diagnostic tests are used to confirm the result of a screening test or, where couples already know that they are carriers of a genetic disorder, to determine as early as possible whether the fetus is affected. These tests will usually be undertaken in a specialist unit where genetic counseling is available. A number of diagnostic tests are undertaken prenatally and all involve the collection of fetal cells. Such tests which require sampling of amniotic fluid (amniocentesis), placenta (chorionic villus sampling, CVS) or fetal blood are necessarily invasive and carry an element of risk.

Couples who are carriers of a genetic disorder will generally be unaware of this until they have an affected child. They will tend to seek prenatal genetic tests in subsequent pregnancies to avoid having a further affected child. Sometimes several pregnancies in a row may be affected, with the accompanying distress of difficult decision making and/or termination of the pregnancy.

Prenatal diagnosis (PND) allows for the detection of genetic disorders. However, the result is sometimes not available until well on into the pregnancy and will always involve the anguishing decision of whether or not to terminate the pregnancy. Preimplantation genetic diagnosis (PGD) has been developed to sample cells from an early in vitro embryo. Affected embryos can then be discarded, allowing the implantation of unaffected embryos. The trauma of termination, or even serial terminations, of pregnancy can be avoided.

Genetic disorders

Genetic disorders fall into two broad categories; chromosomal anomalies and gene defects.

Chromosomal anomalies Chromosomes are the structures in the nucleus of a cell which carry the genes of the individual concerned. Normal human (diploid) cells contain 46 chromosomes – 22 pairs of autosomes and 2 sex chromosomes XX (female) and XY (male). Gametes normally have only 23 chromosomes (22 autosomes and 1 sex chromosome) and are derived from diploid germ cells through a process of reduction division called meiosis. During this process the chromosomes exchange genetic material with their pairs (recombination) and segregate to give rise to haploid gametes with single complements of chromosomes. Sometimes errors occur in this process, giving rise to chromosomal anomalies such as aneuploidies and translocations. Aneuploidies result from failures in segregation resulting in gametes carrying more or fewer chromosomes than normal. Aneuploidies are, for the most part fatal, since embryos carrying only one copy of an autosome cannot survive. Those which do survive with three copies (trisomy) are abnormal. The most common is trisomy of chromosome 21 (Down's syndrome) but trisomies of chromosomes 13 and 18 also occur. Failure of the sex chromosomes to segregate can lead to Klinefelter's syndrome (XXY males) or Turner's syndrome (women with only one X chromosome) which both lead to infertility. Translocations result from errors in recombination where genes are moved to another part of the same chromosome or to a different chromosome and can also result in genetic disorders.

Gene defects

Genes are basic units of genetic material formed of DNA and are usually carried in a particular place on a chromosome. Each gene codes for a particular protein which may be involved in the growth, development, maintenance and reproduction of the organism. In humans genes occur as pairs of alleles on matching chromosomes. Sometimes errors (mutations) may occur in the genetic code which may alter or inhibit the function of the resultant protein. Generally, a defective allele is compensated by its normal pair. However, if these defects are passed down through the germ cells they may lead to serious genetic disease. These diseases may result from single gene defects (monogenic diseases) or from defects in a combination of genes (polygenic diseases). In autosomal recessive diseases, such as cystic fibrosis, ß- thalassemia or sickle cell disease, both alleles have to be affected, i.e. both parents have contributed a defective gene. In X-linked disorders, such as Duchenne's muscular dystrophy, mental retardation and hemophilia the disease is caused in males by a single gene defect on the X-chromosome. Huntington's chorea is an example of a dominant gene defect where only one allele needs to be affected for the disease to occur. This is a late onset disease leading to widespread neuronal degeneration, dementia and death.

Preimplantation genetic diagnosis

Preimplantation genetic diagnosis allows the analysis of the genotype of an embryo prior to implantation. The technique involves the removal of individual cells (blastomeres) from 4 to 8 cell embryos to determine whether or not they are carrying a defective gene or chromosomal anomaly.

The procedure was developed at the Hammersmith Hospital in London some ten years ago[1] using the then novel technique of polymerase chain reaction (PCR) and a probe specific for the Y-chromosome. Since then specific genetic probes for particular disorders have been developed and fluorescence in situ hybridization (FISH) used to determine gender. PGD is now possible for some two dozen genetic disorders but some 200 disorders would be amenable to such diagnosis.

Embryo biopsy

The first stage of PGD involves the removal of one or two blastomeres from an in vitro embryo. One cell is generally taken from a 4 to 6 cell embryo whereas two may safely be taken from an 8 cell embryo. To do this a hole is made in the zona pellucida which surrounds the embryo and a micropipette inserted. The embryo is steadied against a holding pipette and the blastomere aspirated into the micropipette. This provides a miniscule amount of material for analysis compared to that obtained for PND so that the sensitivity and accuracy of the subsequent diagnostic tests are especially important. The embryo is maintained incubation while the diagnostic test is carried out on the isolated blastomere.

Polymerase chain reaction

To detect the presence of one gene in one cell is practically impossible. PCR uses the properties of DNA and enzymes to cut and copy it to amplify the gene which is being sought. After a number of cycles of amplification sufficient DNA from the gene in question is obtained to sequence and analyze it for the presence of mutations.

Fluorescence in situ hybridization

When PGD was first developed, PCR using a Y-specific probe was used to detect the gender of embryos where they were at risk of suffering from an X-linked disease. Male embryos, carrying a Y chromosome identified in this way, would not be implanted. These days FISH would be used to identify male and female embryos. Chromosome specific DNA probes have a fluorescent marker attached, a different color for X and Y, and these are then incubated with the isolated blastomere on a slide. Observation of the resultant colored spots through a fluorescence microscope will identify whether the blastomere comes from a male or female embryo. The technique can also be used to detect aneuploidies.

Availability and success of PGD

Since PGD was introduced a decade ago the number of centers offering a preimplantation genetic diagnostic service has slowly but steadily increased. In the TRAC survey (see chapter 18) 43 respondents said that their clinics were offering or were intending to offer PGD. In 1997 the ESHRE established a PGD Consortium[2] and encouraged active centers to participate. The objectives of the consortium are:

- To survey the availability of PGD for different conditions facilitating cross-referral of patients;
- To collect prospectively and retrospectively data on the accuracy, reliability and effectiveness of PGD;
- To initiate follow-up studies of pregnancies and children born;
- To produce guidelines and recommend PGD protocols to promote best practice;
- To formulate consensus on the use of PGD.

By November 1998 over 25 centers had joined the consortium although only 12 had fulfilled their obligations of membership. These centers had reported 318 referrals for PGD. Although a number were referred for the detection of chromosomal disorders the majority were referred for single gene defects (see tables 3.1 and 3.2 below)

Table 3.1   Cases referred to ESHRE Consortium members for PGD of chromosomal disorders

Type of disorder	Number of referrals
Aneuploidy risk	27
Deletion	3
Inversion	1
Klinefelter syndrome	9
Male meiotic abnormalities	3
Reciprocal translocation	36
Sex chromosome mosaicism	4

The group indicated as 'aneuploidy risk' included patients with previous trisomy or triploidy pregnancies, age related aneuploidy or recurrent abortion. In these cases neither of the two partners had a constitutional chromosmal abnormality. In four cases there was a combination of two indications.

Table 3.2   Cases referred to ESHRE Consortium members for PGD of single gene defects

Genetic Disorder	Number of referrals
ß-thalassemia	12
Charcot-Marie-Tooth disease	11
Cystic fibrosis	30
Cystic fibrosis/CBAVD	8
Gaucher's disease	2
Huntington's chorea	12
Myotonic dystrophy	20
Neurofibromatosis type 1	2
Rhesus-isoimmunisation	3
Sandhoff disease	2
Sickle cell anemia	2
Spinal muscular atrophy	8
Tay-Sachs disease	8
X-linked Becker's muscular dystrophy	9
X-linked Charcot-Marie-Tooth	3
X-linked Coffin-Lowry syndrome	2
X-linked Duchenne muscular dystrophy	20
X-linked FG syndrome	2
X-linked fragile-X	13
X-linked granulomatous disease	2
X-linked hemophilia	14
X-linked hydrocephalus	2
X-linked mental retardation	7
X-linked Wiskott-Aldrich syndrome	5
Unknown	2

There were a further 30 single referrals for different monogenic disorders.

The reasons for referral for PGD were genetic risk and previous termination of pregnancy (89); genetic risk and objection to termination of pregnancy (207); genetic risk and sub- or infertility (99), genetic risk and sterilization (2); age related aneuploidy (19); other (15); unknown (5).

The success rate of PGD in terms of efficiency and accuracy and in live birth rate is largely unknown since insufficient statistics are available. A study from Belgium[3] indicates that in a series of 333 biopsies no diagnosis was possible in 43 (12.9%) because of no amplification, inconsistent results or contamination. The success in terms of pregnancies was 10 out of 61 cycles (16%) or 10 out of 48 transfers (21%). In 1996 world figures for PGD gave a pregnancy rate of 25% per cycle and 29% per transfer.[4]

Preimplantation genetic diagnosis is now available in most European countries. In Germany[5] and Austria[6] the law effectively prohibits PGD since embryos may only be created for the establishment of a pregnancy and therefore cannot be discarded. However, patients from these countries can be referred elsewhere for PGD.

Access, ethics and regulation

With the imminent completion of the Human Genome Project there is likely to be a surge in the understanding of human genetics and the function of human genes. Not only will more genes be identified as being associated with particular diseases, thus enabling earlier diagnosis, but also a greater understanding of gene function will allow the development of therapies for these diseases. As people become more aware of their genotype through the greater availability of commercial diagnostic services the demands for preimplantation diagnosis may increase. This raises a number of issues.

Access to PGD

It was clear from the TRAC survey that PGD is being offered in private as well as public IVF clinics. Given an increase in demand for PGD, this is more likely to be met through the private sector than the public sector because of the costs involved. This may limit some access to those with the means to pay. Currently PGD is offered to individuals at risk of having a child with a serious genetic disorder or chromosomal anomaly. Generally these patients will be referred from genetics centers. However, in the future IVF patients in general and the wider public may also wish to have access to PGD. The time may come where services may wish to limit access to those who are at risk.

Preimplantation genetic screening

One set of patients who might seem to be natural candidates for PGD would be patients seeking IVF treatment. Many of these women will be of the age when they would normally receive antenatal screening for aneuploidies. Preimplantation genetic screening (PGS) of all IVF embryos would increase the chances of pregnancy, since embryos with chromosomal abnormalities are less likely to implant and develop and are a frequent cause of miscarriage, and reduce the likelihood of an affected child being born. This would lead to a significant increase in the success of IVF. It would probably not lead to the elimination of CVS or amniocentesis in these cases, since some patients would prefer to double check, but women would have more confidence in refusing such tests if they did not wish to take the small risk of pregnancy loss. It would also seem to be morally more acceptable to undertake this sort of genetic screening at the preimplantation stage if it avoids the likelihood of a termination of pregnancy.

However, PGS for aneuploidy is still largely experimental. Mosaicism is not uncommon in embryonic cells with some having a normal karyotype while others in the same embryo have chromosomal abnormalities. This could lead to misdiagnosis. It is believed that the abnormal cells in early embryos do not go on to form the embryo proper but become part of the trophoblast and then placenta. Possibly viable embryos might therefore be discarded. An alternative would be to look at the chromosome complement of the polar bodies which are extruded during oocyte maturation as part of the process of meiosis. This would in fact provide a screening process which would ensure that only normal oocytes are used for fertilization. However, it would not overcome the problem of paternal aneuploidies being transferred by sperm. Considerable research is still needed in this area before it becomes common practice.

If PGS were to become a normal procedure for IVF patients this would imply that it should eventually be offered by all clinics. But genetic tests bring with them special counseling needs. Patients would need to be properly informed about the risks both of the procedure, embryo biopsy may have a deleterious effect on the embryo, and of the outlook for the child of different kinds of chromosomal abnormality. Patients should be able to choose whether or not they wish to have an embryo implanted rather than embryos being eliminated from transfer by the clinician because a mild abnormality has been detected.

Restriction of PGD to serious genetic disorders

Some legislation, such as that in Spain and Denmark, specifically approves of PGD for the prevention of serious genetic disease. The problem is that on the matter of seriousness even clinical judgement can be subjective. This could be overcome by having an agreed list of specific conditions which are considered to be serious. However, this need not be prescriptive and should be regularly reviewed. Advances in the understanding of genetic disease, together with advances in somatic cell gene therapy, mean that diseases such a cystic fibrosis might become treatable and PND might then be considered more appropriate. Where the diagnosis of serious genetic disease in cases of known risk is concerned it is probably more appropriate that patients are referred to assisted conception clinics by specialist genetics centers. This would mean that patients would have access to expert genetic advice. Self-referral for PGD and IVF following access to commercial genetic testing should be discouraged.

A number of serious genetic disorders begin later in adult life which means that those who are affected can live normally for a considerable span. There is a debate as to whether PGD is appropriate for these disorders. The patterns of inheritance of these diseases vary. Huntington's disease results from a dominant single gene defect and people inheriting this defect will inevitably go down with the disease although they are likely to have a good 30 years of normal life. On the other hand, carrying a genetic defect which predisposes the carrier towards breast cancer may result in a 40 to 50% lifetime risk of breast cancer. One may consider that in the case of Huntington's disease the inevitable onset of debilitating disease and early death justifies the use of PGD and the discarding of affected embryos. But in the case of the breast cancer gene PND may be more appropriate so that the carrier can be informed and adjust their lifestyle accordingly.

Regulation

Other than in the United Kingdom, where PGD comes under the aegis of the Human Fertilisation and Embryology Authority, there is little formal regulation of PGD in Europe[7] yet provision would appear to be expanding in a rather piecemeal fashion. The formation of the ESHRE PGD Consortium may provide some professional self-regulation, and should eventually provide useful statistical data on referrals and outcomes. But in the area of genetic diagnosis quality assurance is essential. In PGD where so little material is available it is essential that the validity of the tests used is properly established before they are used clinically.   This implies continued embryo research and the accurate assessment of false positive and false negative rates.   A number of countries where PGD is being offered do not allow the creation of embryos for research and do not have the research base to do this.

In this chapter I have barely touched on the ethical issues, a good discussion of these is provided by de Wert[8], but they are many and may increase if the demand for genetic testing increases.   The HFEA has also recognized that PGD is reaching a watershed and, together with the Advisory Committee on Genetic Testing, issued a Consultation Document on Preimplantation Genetic Diagnosis in November 1999.   The results of the consultation have not yet been published but when they are they may provide useful guidelines which might be taken up more generally.

Notes

1   Handyside, A.H., Kontiogianni, E.H., Hardy, K. et al (1990), 'Pregnancies from biopsied human preimplantation embryos sexed by Y-specific DNA amplification', *Nature*, vol. 344, pp. 768-770.

2   Geraedts, J., Handyside, A.H., Harper, J., Liebaers, I. Et al (1999) 'Preimplantation Genetic Diagnosis', *Proceedings of the Second TRAC Workshop,* unpublished.

3   Liebaers, I., Sermon, K., Staessen, C. et al (1999) 'Clinical experience with PID and ICSI' in E.Hildt and S.Graumann (eds), *Genetics in Human Reproduction*, Ashgate Publishing Ltd., Aldershot, pp 3-15.

4   Harper, J. C. (1996) 'Preimplantation diagnosis of inherited disease by embryo biopsy: an update of world figures' *Journal of Assisted Reproduction Genetics*, vol 13 (2), pp. 90-95.

5   Mueller, S. (1997) 'Ethics and the regulation of preimplantation diagnosis in Germany', *Eubios Journal of Asian and International Bioethics*, vol. 7, pp. 5-6.

6   Austrian Act on Procreative Medicine (1992), Section 9 (1), *Official Gazette*, No. 275.

7   Gunning, J., (1999) 'Legal regulations concerning preimplantation diagnosis', in E. Hildt and S. Graumann (eds), *Genetics in Human Reproduction*, Ashgate Publishing Ltd, Aldershot, pp. 261-272.

8   De Wert, G., (1999) 'Ethics of preimplantation diagnosis', in E.Hildt and S Graumann (eds), *Genetics in Human Reproduction*, Ashgate Publishing Ltd., Aldershot, pp. 75-96.

4 Future Directions in Research on Human Embryos

MARTIN H. JOHNSON

Introduction

To claim to know the nature of future discoveries in human embryo research is to misunderstand fundamentally the meaning of the word "discovery". The unknown is simply that - unknown, but it is not necessarily unknowable. Research is the process by which conversion occurs. It would be folly therefore to attempt to describe future research outcomes. However, the objective of this chapter is quite different.

It has been claimed that no further research on human embryos is required: that the moral imperative against such research is so strong that there could not be any outcomes sufficiently advantageous to warrant further research. We have done enough research already, it is argued, to tell us what we need to know. The view that we know all that we need to know is, of course, as misguided as that articulated in the first sentence, since it too assumes that the unknowable cannot possibly be useful. This view has been rejected by those Governments that have passed legislation enabling research.

What I will try to do in this Chapter is to examine some possible new developments in research, based not on crystal ball gazing but on existing knowledge or on our current understanding of areas of ignorance. Under research on human embryos, I include any research on gametes which logically requires or strongly demands that an embryo be created to test the outcome of the gamete manipulation, since under most regulatory regimes, and certainly in the UK (Johnson, 2000), this would count as research on embryos. Because this examination is in no way intended to be comprehensive, the chapter will be organized according to a set of generalized research objectives rather than by particular experiments or techniques. By looking at more general objectives and strategies, and illustrating them with examples, a context or framework for further reflection and development is provided.

In formulating and illustrating these general objectives, I am not suggesting that these research developments *should* occur, or even that it might be considered desirable that they *do* occur. Neither do I have time to consider the deeper ethical implications of each nor their legality in the UK or elsewhere. I omit consideration of research on human embryos in connection with preimplantation genetic diagnosis, non-reproductive cloning and use of embryonic stem cells, each of which is covered elsewhere (see Chapters 2, 3 and 9). Finally, I do not have the space to acknowledge all those published references of interest to the wide range of topics considered. I apologize to those who feel their work should have been referenced, but this review simply cannot be comprehensive and gives illustrative example references.

First, the process by which the categorization of research objective has been organized is summarized. The average live birth rate per treatment cycle of in-vitro fertilization (IVF) initiated has only inched upwards in the UK since reliable data were first recorded (HFEA, 1999). More significantly, the range of live birth rates recorded across different treatment centers is wide, even when adjusted for differences in patient profile (HFEA, 1998). These observations imply that not all clinics are effective in the technical aspects of embryo generation, culture, and placement in the female tract. Two aspects of these processes are susceptible to research on embryos, namely more effectively selecting those embryos (or gametes) with the greatest developmental potential (considered in section 1) and improving or maintaining embryo quality by improving the quality of culture media (section 2). Both of these types of research are extensions of existing traditional practice. A third, more interventionist and therefore contentious approach is research aimed at actively improving the quality of the embryo (section 3). The ability to produce more embryos from an individual or couple might facilitate research generally and offer more reliable and less serially invasive therapy. Research into the production of greater embryo numbers is considered in section 4. New assisted reproductive technologies will each demand validation, and this is the subject of section 5. An altogether different type of research stimulus is the demand for parenthood posed by new patterns of personal and social relationships that differ from the conventional heterosexual partnerships of reproductive age. Such approaches are considered in section 6. Finally, research on embryos to improve implantation success is considered in section 7.

1. Research into methods for more effectively selecting those spermatozoa, oocytes or embryos with the greatest potential for development

Much research work has already taken place attempting to identify non-destructively, and preferably non-invasively or via surrogate indicators, those gametes or embryos that have the greatest potential for development (Van Blerkom, 1997). Examples of criteria already being assessed in research projects include the Hyper Osmotic Swelling (HOS) test for spermatozoa (Hossain et al., 1998), the levels of reactive oxygen species and/or leucocyte contamination in semen in relation to the fertilizing ability of spermatozoa (Moilanen et al., 1998), features of spermatozoal maturation such as chromatin packing (Filatov et al., 1999), blood flow to the growing follicle in relation to oocyte potential (Van Blerkom, 1998; Bhal et al., 1999; Coulam et al., 1999), indicators of oocyte well-being derived from measurements on follicular cells (e.g. Stewart and VandeVoort, 1999), free radical production in the insemination drop and ways to reduce the possible adverse effects of large numbers of spermatozoa (Dirnfeld et al., 1999), location and size of pronuclei (Tesarik and Greco, 1999), blastomere morphology (such as fragmentation, relative blastomere size and/or division rate, cytoplasmic granularity etc: Antczak and Van Blerkom, 1999; Van Royen et al., 1999), metabolic activity (Turner et al., 1994) or cytokine production (Kowalik et al., 1999), the use of a biopsied blastomere to measure developmental progress as a surrogate marker for the residual embryo (Geber and Sampaio, 1999) or on which to undertake invasive assays for molecular markers of normal development (e.g. Steuerwald et al., 1999), and the ability to survive in vitro to form a blastocyst (and factors affecting this ability: Rijnders and Jansen, 1999; Jones and Trounson, 1999). Undoubtedly new criteria will be developed and applied, and the existing ones refined and combined, to improve overall the capacity of embryologists to identify more reliably developmental potential or lack of it. For example, as more vital dyes are developed, and more sensitive detection systems used to visualize their emissions, the intracellular concentration of dye required for measurement of both its quantity and its distribution will reduce and the dangers of toxicity recede. This will open increasingly the possibility of measurements being made within a single live oocyte or zygote of, for example, pH, the concentrations of ions, individual proteins or even mRNAs, and of organelles (for example see Sutovsky et al., 1999). This information might then provide useful predictive markers of the developmental potential of the gamete or zygote, something which is clearly needed (Devreker et al., 1999a).

2. Improving embryo quality by improving the quality of culture media

Attempts to develop effective culture media lay at the heart of much of the early work leading to in-vitro fertilization and culture of mammalian embryos. Success was remarkably recent and remains elusive for embryos of most species (Biggers, 1998). This sort of research continues and is still required for human embryos, whether through comparison of different complex media (Conaghan et al., 1998; Karamalegos and Bolton, 1999), sequential use of different media (Pickering et al., 1995; Gardner et al., 1998; Fong and Bongso, 1999), and/or by systematic variation of individual components such as metabolic substrates and growth factors (Coates et al., 1999; Kaye and Gardner, 1999; Sjöblom et al., 1999; Devreker et al., 1999b). In this context, it is important to remember that media do not replicate the conditions encountered by the embryo *in vivo* (Leese, 1998). Rather, media are developed empirically to provide a minimum sustaining environment, all components of which will (ideally) be identified and controlled for purity. Thus, use of media containing complex natural sources of macro-molecules, such as plasma, cell mono-layers, or body secretions (Fong and Bongso, 1999; Ali et al., 2000), is increasingly unacceptable because of the risks of cross-contamination of the embryos with infectious agents. Research to understand the macromolecular requirements of the embryo is still necessary (Gardner et al., 1999).

So all media currently in use require the embryo to adapt to its new artificial environment, and there is clear evidence from study of mouse embryos in vitro that it responds to this environment by modifying its metabolism, its pattern of gene expression, and its chromosomal imprinting status (reviewed Johnson and Nasr-Esfahani, 1994). Many of these adaptive responses are typically stress reactions. Some of these responses may have enduring consequences for the embryo/fetus leading to its death or to effects on the new born. For example, in farm animals in vitro conceptuses produce larger offspring when reimplanted *in utero* (Walker et al., 1996), and whilst there is no evidence that the same applies to human embryos in vitro, future research may reveal whether the longer periods being spent in vitro associated with blastocyst transfer lead to this or other effects. In humans, an effect of maternal diet on the subsequent health of the offspring into adulthood has been proposed (Barker, 1994, 1997; Paneth and Susser, 1995; Paneth et al., 1996; see Johnson, 1999 for discussion), and research to determine when these effects operate during pregnancy and whether known metabolic adaptations to in vitro culture might induce them will be important.

It is not at present clear what part of the relatively low birth rate per cycle of treatment initiated is due to the inadequacy of media currently in use, but it is plausible to believe that further research into the development of media will improve outcome rates. In mice, for example, a retardation in cytokine expression patterns shown by embryos cultured in vitro was at least partially reversed by manipulation of the medium composition (Stojanov et al., 1999).

Attempts to mature oocytes in vitro (see section 4 below) will also succeed or founder in large part on the quality of the media developed.

3. Research to actively improve the quality of the embryo

This approach is more interventionist and therefore more controversial. It accepts that some embryos may be sub-optimal (for example, for reasons of maternal age, follicular pathology, spermatozoal damage etc) but tries to improve survival not by prevention but by correction or amelioration of deficiencies.

Cytoplasmic therapy

The zygote inherits more than a set of chromosomes from each parent. Thus, we inherit from our mothers, but NOT from our fathers, an additional set of replicating chromosomes essential for development in our mitochondria. Mitochondria are responsible for generation of cellular energy and are all received exclusively from the mother via the oocyte. Within each mitochondrion is a small subset of genes on a mitochondrial chromosome. The expression of these genes contributes to mitochondrial replication and function, and, where there are significant accumulations of mitochondrial mutations, to mitochondrial malfunctions. There is evidence that mitochondrial mutations may contribute to oocyte and zygote loss in humans (Barritt et al., 1999). In rarer cases of mothers with diagnosed mitochondrial disease, all her offspring regardless of their sex tend to become diseased. In situations of mitochondrial mutation or disease, the transfer of the pronuclei to a non-affected enucleated ooplasm, or of non-affected ooplasm containing mitochondria to an afflicted oocyte/zygote, might overcome this problem for the children.

Second, the father via the spermatozoon, but NOT in humans the mother, also contributes an essential organelle called the centrosome, which controls how the cells of the conceptus and adult divide and proliferate (Simerly et al., 1995). The centrosome does not have any associated DNA (genes), and thus it is not a genetic component. However, it does replicate and distribute its progeny at division during cycles of cell proliferation, and it does so (usually) in parallel with the nuclear chromosomes. Indeed, without this paternal centrosome, sustained embryonic cell division and proliferation and correct chromosomal segregation do not occur and pregnancy fails. It is possible that spermatozoa from some men have defective centrosomes, which might be "cured" by transferring a pure centrosome from a non-affected individual (but see Moomjy et al., 1999). Considerable research is needed to test and validate such an approach.

Third, the oocyte brings to the conceptus not simply its chromosomes, both nuclear and mitochondrial, but a set of cytoplasmic organelles (other than a centrosome) plus reservoirs of messenger RNA and protein that are essential for the early development of the conceptus up to at least the time of implantation. It has been proposed that any deficiencies in this cytoplasm might be remedied by cytoplasmic transfer of cytoplasm from "good" oocytes (Cohen et al., 1998). For example, oocytes seem to be less viable with increasing time post-ovulation or when taken from older women (Winston et al., 1993). Use of ooplasmic transfer from freshly ovulated oocytes taken from young women might "freshen" them up. Some women may generate large amounts of free oxygen radicals during oogenesis and the damage done to the cytoplasm might likewise be repaired or ameliorated by ooplasmic transfer. It is possible, though unlikely, that the use of non-human ooplasm might be effective therapy for deficiencies in some of the above non-genetic inheritances.

As we understand more about the specific molecular requirements for development, and the consequences of their deficiency, the use of episomal plasmid vectors to drive transient expression of specific genes (or 'anti-genes' for their neutralization) may become a feasible form of therapy. Clearly, much research will be needed to achieve this.

Gene therapy

Defective chromosomal genetic material could lead to embryo or fetal failure or abnormality in the offspring. Current approaches stress selection of embryos not carrying the genetic defect in a form that is expressed (see Chapter 3). Germ line gene therapy, in which the defective gene is replaced, could only be achieved currently through the use of embryonic stem cells (see Chapter 9), since the defective gene in the oocyte/embryo cannot be reliably targeted for replacement. Technological improvements to the frequency of successful gene targeting might change this. Alternatively, it may also be the case that certain defects, expressed relatively early in development, could be overcome by the transfer and expression of episomal DNA, or even of mRNA (Weber et al., 1999), to the zygote to give transient expression for sufficiently long to allow embryo survival.

4. Research into the production of more embryos

Treatment cycles may fail because there are no gametes, no embryos formed from gametes, or too few embryos, necessitating several rounds of patient stimulation and oocyte recovery. Any development that enabled all the gametes that a couple were ever likely to need to be collected in one operation and stored for use would revolutionize treatment and reduce costs. It would also have other potential benefits for research and for tissue therapy.

In-vitro maturation of oocytes

The size of the cohort of oocytes recovered from mature ovarian follicles after hormonal priming using exogenous hormones is variable and limited. Harvesting ovarian oocytes from immature antral, preantral or even primordial follicles followed by their in vitro culture in isolated follicles, in sections of ovary or after isolation as oocytes could potentially produce larger numbers of mature oocytes for use by the oocyte producer herself, for donation, or for research. In addition, the ability to produce large numbers of oocytes, would mean that embryos created from them could be frozen and then thawed and transferred one at a time, so leading to a reduction in multiple pregnancy rates. However, oocyte maturation involves a complex process of cytoplasmic and chromosomal change that has proved difficult to capture in vitro to the point where a high proportion of fully viable oocytes is achieved consistently in any species (Fulka et al., 1998). Recent research in which media, media components and culture conditions are varied has lead to progress in some species (e.g. De La Fuente et al., 1999), including limited progress in primates (Schramm and Bavister, 1999; Mikkelsen et al., 1999; De Vos et al., 1999; Cobo et al., 1999), and this area undoubtedly represents a major area for continuing research. In addition to the technological aspects of improving the yield of viable oocytes, it will also be necessary for research to address issues of oocyte normality. A better understanding of the in vitro conditions that facilitate oocyte maturation may also shed light on the causes of infertility or of inferior embryo production arising from abnormal maturation *in vivo* and so might offer ways to improve maturation *in situ*.

Use of cadavers and fetuses as a source of oocytes

An alternative source of oocytes is the ovaries from women who die young or from fetuses. Techniques for harvesting these oocytes would need to be developed, as would in vitro maturation schedules (see Section 4i). There are major ethical issues to be resolved, particularly with regard to consent, and these, rather than technical difficulties, form the main stumbling block additional to those inherent in in vitro culture.

Use of ES cells as a source of gametes

An alternative strategy to ovarian harvesting would be to try and induce human embryonal stem cells (Pera et al., 2000 and Chapter 9) to differentiate into gametes in vitro. Stem cells have the potential to produce gametes - this is integral to their definition as totipotent. Research to determine how to achieve the production of gametes in vitro would be needed. If combined with somatic cell nuclear transfer into the ES cells (Wilmut et al., 1997), such an approach could produce gametes with the same genetic make up as the infertile person which, if their infertility was not itself genetically based, would permit them to parent a genetically related child.

Making human gametes in living incubators

Alternatively, in individuals who had germ stem cells but in whom germ cell maturation failed, the stem cells might be transplanted into the gonads of immuno-incompetent animals such as athymic mice (Dobrinski et al., 1999; Ogawa et al., 2000). If the failure of the germ cells to develop in the donor gonad had been due to some feature of the gonad rather than an inherent deficiency in the germ cell itself, the spermatozoa or oocytes produced in the mice might be harvestable for use. Issues of xeno-transplantation arise with such an approach.

Inducing cells to undergo meiosis in vitro

Rather than actually trying to make mature gametes in vitro or in living incubators, an alternative approach might be to develop in-vitro systems to simply induce meiotic divisions in cells. Although germ stem cells would be an obvious starting point for this work, the demonstration through Dolly that nuclei from differentiated cells can under the right conditions express toti-potentiality might mean that any cell, if exposed to the appropriate in vitro conditions, could be induced to enter meiosis so generating a haploid chromosomal product or "pronucleus" which could then be injected into an enucleated carrier oocyte.

In-vitro maturation of spermatids

In azoospermic men in which elongated spermatids have not been observed, there remains a belief that round spermatids can be recovered and used in ICSI. However, the difficulty in recognizing round spermatids (Sutovsky et al., 1999) and then isolating them (Lassalle et al., 1999), and the low efficiency of their use for generating pregnancy (Prapas et al., 1999) has lead to the suggestion that in vitro culture systems for spermatids (and perhaps ultimately for spermatocytes) might provide a more effective route to fertility treatment for such men.

Gamete cryopreservation

Oocyte cryopreservation would be a useful adjunct to many of the above techniques, as would the more efficient cryo-storage of spermatozoa (Morris et al., 1999). The former has been achieved in mice (George et al., 1994), but only episodically in humans, although a fully successful and reliable regime must be near with further research (Gook and Edgar, 1999). In addition, the ability to freeze oocytes would mean that eggs could be fertilized one at a time and so lead to a reduction in multiple pregnancy rates.

Embryo splitting

The production of multiple embryos from a single zygote by embryo splitting in vitro is currently limited to a maximum of between two and four. This approach has recently been reported to result in live young in the rhesus monkey (Chan et al., 2000b), although in other species it has been achievable for some time. There is a limit of 2-4 because there appears to be a set number of cleavage divisions that is characteristic for the species after which the initiation of cell differentiation into trophoblast and pluriblast occurs (Ziomek and Johnson, 1981; Johnson, 1996; Johnson and Selwood, 1996). If a single embryo is split into too many parts, then there are simply not sufficient cells in each part to make both pluriblast and trophoblast in adequate amounts, usually the crucial deficiency being in the pluriblast. In consequence, a blastocyst without developmental potential forms. If the timing of the differentiative initiation could be controlled and delayed, then each embryo could be grown and split *ad infinitum*, thereby producing multiple copies. The signal to differentiate could then be given, so yielding multiple blastocysts for transfer, constituting a clone of genetically identical embryos. One could then be transferred during a natural cycle, and, if pregnancy did not result, repeat transfers of single blastocysts could be undertaken until pregnancy occurred. This scenario provides minimal risk of hyperstimulation and multiple pregnancy with multiple opportunities to produce the "same genetic baby", which may itself have a strong appeal to prospective parents. The remaining blastocysts could then be stored as a tissue bank reserve for the child to be. Understanding the basis for the timing of the earliest differentiative event might also have benefits for understanding and controlling certain cancers of the early embryo and trophoblast.

This approach, if combined with more successful gene targeting techniques (see 3ii above), might also facilitate curative therapies for improvement of embryo genetic quality.

5. Validating new assisted conception methodologies

It would be foolish to believe that all novel technologies for the alleviation of infertility have been described, or variations of existing ones exhausted. For each novel technology, the question will arise: is it a valid option and what is its reliability? The comparison will always have to be with well established existing methods, and, just as ICSI is still being compared with

IVF (Staessen et al., 1999) and cryopreserved with fresh embryos (Aytoz et al., 1999), each new technology will require a set of research protocols involving the use of human embryos.

6. Providing new technological routes to parenthood to satisfy new patterns of parenting

As social patterns of partnership change, so social patterns of parenthood are changing (Johnson, 1999). Thus not only are post-reproductive age heterosexual partnerships and individuals desiring reproductive options, but individuals and same sex couples are likewise wishing to express themselves or their mutual commitment reproductively. In particular, given the heavy emphasis in our contemporary culture on the importance of genetics (Johnson, 1997), an approximately equivalent genetic contribution from both parenting partners may be desired. However, in humans (mammals) sexual reproduction is obligatory because the genetic contributions from the mother and the father, whilst being as it were anatomically equivalent (equal numbers of chromosomes from each) are not functionally equivalent. This is because a subset of genes is modified epigenetically (imprinted) during spermatozoal and oocyte formation (Surani, 1999). An epigenetic change does not affect the actual nucleotide base composition of the genes (the 'genetic code' itself), but does affect the way in which the genes in the imprinted subset are 'wrapped up' in proteins. Moreover, it does so in a way that is perpetuated each time the genes are replicated during cell proliferation: it is an inherited epigenetic imprint. This imprinting process affects the availability for expression of these genes during embryogenic, embryonic and fetal development and, indeed adult life. Thus, the imprinted genes may never be expressed, or may be expressed in reduced amounts or at different times from the non-imprinted genes. Because the subset of genes which is modified epigenetically during oocyte formation is different from the subset modified during spermatozoal formation, so-called "parental specific imprinting" of genes, sexual reproduction is obligatory in mammals (Johnson, 1999). Thus, in order to have the complete set of functional genes required for full development a conceptus must receive one set from mother and one set from father: two sets from father or two sets from mother (both of which situations can be achieved experimentally) results in failure of the conceptus to complete development. Ways to overcome or circumvent the effects of parental imprinting might be the subject of embryo research, as might other ways of achieving a balanced genetic contribution from each same sex parent.

Tetra-parentage

An approach which circumvents, rather than overcomes, the effects of parental imprinting has long been available in mice (McLaren, 1978) and there seems no clear reason technically why it should not also work in humans. A gay man and a lesbian could conceive through IVF to produce embryos containing chromosomes derived from each in equal proportions, and the gay man's male partner likewise could conceive with the lesbian's female partner. If one embryo from each IVF procedure were then taken and the two aggregated together, a tetra-parental embryo with approximately equal genetic contributions from each of the four parents would result. It would be necessary to make sure that both embryos making up the aggregate were of the same sex, otherwise hermaphoditism in the off-spring might occur. This could be achieved by pre-implantation testing of each of the embryos to be aggregated for sex. It would also be necessary to demonstrate that cells from both of the aggregated embryos contributed significant numbers of cells to the pluriblast of the inner cell mass from which the embryo proper (rather than the placenta) is derived, otherwise all of the cells of one embryo might go to the placenta (Johnson, 1996; Johnson and Selwood, 1996). By such a route, an approximate equivalence of genetic parenting between partners might be achieved, and the feasibility of such an approach could be confirmed through embryo research.

Such a multi-parental approach need not of course be limited to the homosexual community - a group of people each wishing to have a genetic input into a single off-spring could use the same approach, for example one male and two female genetic parents, or a commune of genetic parents. However, there is an upper limit to the number of embryos that can be aggregated and all still contribute significantly to the off-spring. In practice, no more than two to three aggregated embryos (i.e. a maximum of four to six genetic parents) is likely to be successful, but this could be determined and possibly manipulated as an outcome of research.

Imprinting

The objective of research on imprinting would be to investigate the molecular basis of the imprinting process (Surani, 1999), the time at which during gametogenesis and early development key imprinting events occur (Kato et al., 1999; Shamanski et al., 1999), and how they could be manipulated successfully. For example, it might prove possible to take the male pronucleus and pass it, via a nuclear transfer technique, through female cytoplasm in a germ cell to change the imprint to that of a female. It could then be transferred to an oocyte with a second male pronucleus that had not been so treated to produce a zygote capable of development, but with two male genetic parents. The reverse might become possible with female pronuclei. By such a route the requirement for one male and one female genetic parent would be circumvented.

Unconventional patterns of pregnancy

The possibility of carrying a pregnancy at a site other than the uterus might be a legitimate area of research to help women with no or an abnormal uterus, or men. Fetal survival at such sites can occur but is rare (Ludwig et al., 1999) and usually dangerous to the health of the pregnant woman and her fetus. Research into in vitro systems for developing the fetus would achieve similar ends. The most difficult period for development in vitro is probably that which spans the early embryogenic and embryonic phases of development (Johnson and Everitt, 2000). In such work, it is important to be aware that recent research on development *in vivo* is suggesting that traits (physical, behavioural, pathological) thought previously to be unaffected by intra-uterine experiences are now being shown to be influenced by them (reviewed in Johnson, 1999). Use of surrogate sites for development might therefore enhance development or exacerbate any adverse effects of intra-uterine life. This problem is similar to that raised by the much shorter periods in vitro experienced during IVF (see section 2 above).

7. Improving implantation through research on human embryos

Zona methods

Implantation can fail if the zona pellucida surrounding the embryo fails to lyse, perhaps because it has been made resistant by in vitro conditions ("hardened"). Existing research aims to either prevent zona hardening or to circumvent it using physical, chemical or laser treatment to make a hole in the zona. Further developments in this area are possible, although likely to be largely of a technical nature.

Embryo methods

A different approach might be the transfer to zygotes of mRNA, or of DNA constructs using an appropriate early expressing promoter, to enable transient expression of proteins that facilitated zona lysis or attachment. Such constructs might be injected, transfected (by lipofection or viral vector) or carried in on spermatozoa, as has already been demonstrated to be possible for primates (Chan et al., 2000a). Alternatively, embryos might be pre-treated chemically with agents that enhanced their ability to interact with the endometrium through the promotion of cytokine activity or responsiveness.

Conclusions

Since the original research on human oocytes and embryos by Edwards and his colleagues that led to IVF, research has continued to expand the practical and conceptual possibilities for regulating fertility and manipulating reproductive outcomes. These changing practices and possibilities have themselves changed social attitudes and challenged ethical thinking. The impact of these emergent technologies on attitudes to gender, sexuality, the nature of the family, and the relative roles of inheritance, intra-uterine environment and post-natal experience on the development of human traits has been and continues to be profound. As said at the outset, the scenarios used to illustrate possible directions of future research on human embryos or on the fertilization process itself are neither exhaustive nor obligatory. Many of them may seem alien, some may seem legitimate. It was not the purpose of this chapter to make these distinctions but simply to provide illustrations of the range of possibilities we may encounter in the near future.

References

Ali, J., Shahata, M.A.M. and Al-Natsha, S.D. (2000), 'Formulation of a protein-free medium for human assisted reproduction', *Human Reproduction,* vol. 5, pp. 145-156.

Antczak, M. and Van Blerkom, J. (1999), 'Temporal and spatial aspects of fragmentation in early human embryos: possible effects on developmental competence and association with the differential elimination of regulatory proteins from polarized domains', *Human Reproduction*, vol. 14, pp. 429-47.

Aytoz, A., Van den Abbeel, E., Bonduelle, M., Camus, M., Joris, H., Van Steirteghem, A. and Devroey, P. (1999), 'Obstetric outcome of pregnancies after the transfer of cryopreserved and fresh embryos obtained by conventional in-vitro fertilization and intracytoplasmic spermatozoal injection', *Human Reproduction*, vol. 14, pp. 2619-2624.

Barker, D.J.P. (1994), *Mothers, babies and disease in later life*, BMJ Publishing Group, London.

Barker, D.J.P. (1997), 'The fetal origins of coronary heart disease', *Acta Paediatrica*, Supplement 422, pp.78-82.

Barritt, J.A., Brenner, C.A., Cohen, J. and Matt, D.W. (1999), 'Mitochondrial DNA rearrangements in human oocytes and embryos', *Molecular Human Reproduction*, vol. 5, pp. 927-933.

Bhal, P.S., Pugh, N.D., Chui, D.K., Gregory, L., Walker, S.M. and Shaw, R.W. (1999), 'The use of transvaginal power Doppler ultrasonography to evaluate the relationship between perifollicular vascularity and outcome in in-vitro fertilization treatment cycles', *Human Reproduction*, vol. 14, pp. 939-945.

Biggers, J.D. (1998), 'Reflections on the culture of the preimplantation embryo', *Internatiuonal Journal of Developmental Biology*, vol. 42, pp. 879-84.

Chan, A.W.S., Luetjens, C.M., Dominko, T., Ramalho-Santos, J., Simerly, C.R., Hewitson, L. and Schatten, G. (2000a), 'Foreign DNA transmission by ICSI: injection of spermatozoa bound with exogenous DNA results in embryonic GFP expression and live Rhesus monkey births', *Molecular Human Reproduction*, vol. 6, pp. 26-33.

Chan, A.W., Dominko, T., Luetjens, C.M., Neuber, E., Martinovich, C., Hewitson, L., Simerly, C.R. and Schatten, G.P. (2000b), 'Clonal Propagation of Primate Offspring by Embryo Splitting', *Science*, vol. 287, pp. 317-319.

Coates, A., Rutherford, A.J., Hunter, H. and Leese, H.J. (1999), 'Glucose-free medium in human in vitro fertilization and embryo transfer: a large-scale, prospective, randomized clinical trial', *Fertility and Sterility*, vol. 72, pp. 229-32.

Cobo, A.C., Requena, A., Neuspiller, F., Aragonés, M., Mercader, A., Navarro, J., Simón, C., Remohí, J. and Pellicer, A. (1999), 'Maturation in vitro of human oocytes from unstimulated cycles: selection of the optimal day for ovum retrieval based on follicular size', *Human Reproduction*, vol. 14, pp. 1864-1868.

Cohen, J., Scott R., Alikani, M., Schimmel, T., Munne, S., Levron, J., Wu, L., Brenner, C., Warner, C. and Willadsen, S. (1998), 'Ooplasmic transfer in mature human oocytes', *Molecular Human Reproduction*, vol. 4, pp. 269-280.

Conaghan, J., Hardy, K., Leese, H.J., Winston, R.M. and Handyside, A.H. (1998), 'Culture of human preimplantation embryos to the blastocyst stage: a comparison of 3 media', *International Journal of Developmental Biology*, vol. 42, pp. 885-93.

Coulam, C.B., Goodman, C. and Rinehart, J.S. (1999), 'Colour Doppler indices of follicular blood flow as predictors of pregnancy after in-vitro fertilization and embryo transfer', *Human Reproduction*, vol. 14, pp. 1979-1982.

De La Fuente, R., O'Brien, M.J. and Eppig, J.J. (1999), 'Epidermal growth factor enhances preimplantation developmental competence of maturing mouse oocytes', *Human Reproduction*, vol. 14, pp. 3060-3068.

De Vos, A., Van de Velde, H., Joris, H. and Van Steirteghem, A. (1999), 'In-vitro matured metaphase-I oocytes have a lower fertilization rate but similar embryo quality as mature metaphase-II oocytes after intracytoplasmic spermatozoal injection', *Human Reproduction*, vol. 14, pp. 1859-1863.

Devreker, F., Pogonici, E., De Maertelaer, V., Revelard, P., Van den Bergh, M. and Englert, Y. (1999a), 'Selection of good embryos for transfer depends on embryo cohort size: implications for the 'mild ovarian stimulation' debate', *Human Reproduction*, vol. 14, pp. 3002-3008.

Devreker, F., Van den Bergh, M., Biramane, J., Winston, R.M.L., Englert, Y. and Hardy, K. (1999b), 'Effects of taurine on human embryo development in vitro', *Human Reproduction*, vol. 14, pp. 2350-2356.

Dirnfeld, M., Bider, D., Koifman, M., Calderon, I. and Abramovici, H. (1999), 'Shortened exposure of oocytes to spermatozoa improves in-vitro fertilization outcome: a prospective, randomized, controlled study', *Human Reproduction*, vol. 14, pp. 2562-2564.

Dobrinski, I., Avarbock, M.R. and Brinster, R.L. (1999), 'Transplantation of germ cells from rabbits and dogs into mouse testes', *Biology of Reproduction*, vol. 61, pp. 1331-1339.

Filatov, M.V., Semenova, E.V., Vorob'eva, O.A., Leont'eva, O.A. and Drobchenko, E.A. (1999), 'Relationship between abnormal spermatozoal chromatin packing and IVF results', *Molecular Human Reproduction*, vol. 5, pp. 825-830.

Fong, C.-Y. and Bongso, A. (1999), 'Comparison of human blastulation rates and total cell number in sequential culture media with and without co-culture', *Human Reproduction*, vol. 14, pp. 774-781.

Fulka, J. Jr., First, N.L. and Moor, R.M. (1998), 'Nuclear and cytoplasmic determinants involved in the regulation of mammalian oocyte maturation', *Molecular Human Reproduction*, vol. 4, pp. 41-49.

Gardner, D.K., Rodriegez-Martinez, H. and Lane, M. (1999), 'Fetal development after transfer is increased by replacing protein with the glycosaminoglycan hyaluronan for mouse embryo culture and transfer', *Human Reproduction*, vol. 14, pp. 2575-2580.

Gardner, D.K., Schoolcraft, W.B., Wagley, L. et al. (1998), 'A prospective randomized trial of blastocyst culture and transfer in in-vitro fertilization', *Human Reproduction*, vol. 13, pp. 3434-3440.

Geber, S. and Sampaio, M. (1999), 'Blastomere development after embryo biopsy: a new model to predict embryo development and to select for transfer', *Human Reproduction*, vol. 14, pp. 782-786.

George, M.A., Johnson, M.H. and Howlett, S.K. (1994), 'Assessment of the developmental potential of frozen-thawed mouse oocytes', *Human Reproduction*, vol. 9, pp. 130-136.

Gook, D.A. and Edgar, D.H. (1999), 'Cryopreservation of the human female gamete: current and future issues', *Human Reproduction*, vol. 14, pp. 2938-2940.

HFEA (1998), *Patient's Guide to DI and IVF Clinics*, Human Fertilisation and Embryology Authority, 30 Artillery Lane, London E1 7LS.

HFEA (1999), *Annual Report*, Human Fertilisation and Embryology Authority, Paxton House, 30 Artillery Lane, London E1 7LS.
http://www.hfea.gov.uk/frame3.htm

Hossain, A.M., Rizk, B., Barik, S., Huff, C. and Thorneycroft, I.H. (1998), 'Time course of hypo-osmotic swellings of human spermatozoa: evidence of ordered transition between swelling subtypes', *Human Reproduction*, vol. 13, pp. 1578-83.

Johnson, M.H. (1996), 'The origins of pluriblast and trophoblast in the eutherian conceptus', *Reproduction, Fertility and Development*, vol. 8, pp. 699-709.

Johnson, M.H. (1997), 'Genetics, the free market and reproductive medicine', *Human Reproduction*, vol. 12, pp. 408-410.

Johnson, M.H. (1999), 'A biomedical perspective on parenthood', in A. Bainham, S.D. Sclater and M. Richards (eds.), *What is a parent? A Socio-legal Analysis*, Hart Publishing Ltd., Oxford and Portland, pp. 47-71.

Johnson, M.H. (2000), 'The regulation of human embryo research in the UK: what are the implications for therapeutic research?', in J. Gunning (ed.), *Assisted Conception: Research, Ethics and Law*, Ashgate Publishing, pp. 117-126.

Johnson, M.H. and Everitt, B.J. (2000), *Essential Reproduction*, 5th Edition, Blackwell Science, Oxford.

Johnson, M.H. and Nasr-Esfahani, M.H. (1994), 'Radical solutions and cultural problems', *BioEssays*, vol. 16, pp. 31-38.

Johnson, M.H. and Selwood, L. (1996), 'The nomenclature of early development in mammals', *Reproduction, Fertility and Development*, vol. 8, pp.759-764.

Jones, G.M. and Trounson, A.O. (1999), 'The benefits of extended culture', *Human Reproduction*, vol. 14, pp. 1405-1408.

Karamalegos, C. and Bolton, V.N. (1999), 'A prospective comparison of 'in house' and commercially prepared Earle's balanced salt solution in human in-vitro fertilization', *Human Reproduction*, vol. 14, pp. 1842-1846.

Kato, Y., Rideout, W.M., Hilton, K., Barton, S.C., Tsunoda, Y. and Surani, M.A. (1999), 'Developmental potential of mouse primordial germ cells', *Development*, vol. 126, pp. 1823-32.

Kaye, P.L. and Gardner, H.G. (1999), 'Preimplantation access to maternal insulin and albumin increases fetal growth rate in mice', *Human Reproduction*, vol. 14, pp. 3052-3059.

Kowalik, A., Liu, H.-C., He, Z.-Y., Mele, C., Barmat, L. and Rosenwaks, Z. (1999), 'Expression of the insulin-like growth factor-1 gene and its receptor in preimplantation mouse embryos; is it a marker of embryo viability? ', *Molecular Human Reproduction*, vol. 5, pp. 861-865.

Lassalle, B., Ziyyat, A., Testart, J., Finaz, C. and Lefèvre, A. (1999), 'Flow cytometric method to isolate round spermatids from mouse testis', *Human Reproduction*, vol. 14, pp. 388-394.

Leese, H.J. (1998), 'Human embryo culture: back to nature', *Journal of Assisted Reproduction and Genetics*, vol. 15, pp. 466-468.

Ludwig, M., Kaisi, M., Bauer, O. and Diedrich, K. (1999), 'Case Report: The forgotten child— a case of heterotopic, intra-abdominal and intrauterine pregnancy carried to term', *Human Reproduction*, vol. 14, pp. 1372-1374.

McLaren, A. (1975), 'Sex chimaerism and germ cell distribution in a series of chimaeric mice', *Journal of Embryology and Experimental Morphology*, vol. 33, pp. 205-216.

Mikkelsen, A.L., Smith, S.D. and Lindenberg, S. (1999), 'In-vitro maturation of human oocytes from regularly menstruating women may be successful without follicle stimulating hormone priming', *Human Reproduction*, vol. 14, pp. 1847-1851.

Moilanen, J.M., Carpen, O. and Hovatta, O. (1998), 'Flow cytometric light scattering analysis, acrosome reaction, reactive oxygen species production and leukocyte contamination of semen preparation in prediction of fertilization rate in vitro', *Human Reproduction*, vol. 13, pp. 2568-2574.

Moomjy, M., Colombero, L.T., Veeck, L.L., Rosenwaks, Z. and Palermo, G.D. (1999), 'Sperm integrity is critical for normal mitotic division and early embryonic development', *Molecular Human Reproduction*, vol. 5, pp. 836-844.

Morris, G.J., Acton, E. and Avery, S. (1999), 'A novel approach to sperm cryopreservation', *Human Reproduction*, vol. 14, pp. 1013-1021.

Ogawa, T., Dobrinski, I., Avarbock, M.R. and Brinster, R.L. (2000), 'Transplantation of male germ line stem cells restores fertility in infertile mice', *Nature Medicine*, vol. 6, pp. 29-34.

Paneth, N. and Susser, M. (1995), 'Early origin of coronary heart disease (the "Barker hypothesis")', *British Medical Journal*, vol. 310, pp. 411-412.

Paneth, N., Ahmed, F. and Stein, D.S. (1996), 'Early nutritional origins of hypertension: a hypothesis still lacking support', Journal of Hypertension, vol. 14, pp. S121-129.

Pera, M.F., Reubinoff, B. and Trounson, A. (2000), 'Human embryonic stem cells', *Journal of Cell Science*, vol. 113, pp. 5-10.

Pickering, S.J., Taylor, A., Johnson, M.H. and Braude, P.R. (1995), 'An analysis of multi-nucleated blastomere formation in human embryos', *Human Reproduction*, vol 10, pp. 1912-1922.

Prapas, Y., Chatziparasidou, A., Vanderzwalmen, P., Nijs, M., Prapas, N., Lejeune, B., Vlassis, G. and Schoysman, R. (1999), 'Spermatid injection: Reconsidering spermatid injection', *Human Reproduction*, vol. 14, pp. 2186-2188.

Rijnders, P.M. and Jansen, C.A.M. (1999), 'Influence of group culture and culture volume on the formation of human blastocysts: a prospective randomized study', *Human Reproduction*, vol. 14, pp. 2333-2337.

Schramm, R.D. and Bavister, B.D. (1999), 'A macaque model for studying mechanisms controlling oocyte development and maturation human and non-human primates', *Human Reproduction*, vol. 14, pp. 2544-2555.

Shamanski, F.L., Kimura, Y., Lavoir, M.-C., Pedersen, R.A. and Yanagimachi, R. (1999), 'Status of genomic imprinting in mouse spermatids', *Human Reproduction*, vol. 14, pp. 1050-1056.

Simerly, C., Wu, G., Ord, T., et al. (1995), 'The paternal inheritance of the centrosome, the cells microtubule-organising centre, in humans, and the implications for infertility', *Nature Medicine*, vol 1, pp. 47-52.

Sjöblom, C., Wikland, M. and Robertson, S.A. (1999), 'Granulocyte–macrophage colony-stimulating factor promotes human blastocystdevelopment in vitro', *Human Reproduction*, vol. 14, pp. 3069-3076.

Staessen, C., Camus, M., Clasen, K., De Vos, A. and Van Steirteghem, A. (1999), 'Conventional in-vitro fertilization versus intracytoplasmic sperm injection in sibling oocytes from couples with tubal infertility and normozoospermic semen', *Human Reproduction*, vol. 14, pp. 2474-2479.

Steuerwald, N., Cohen, J., Herrera, R.J. and Brenner, C.A. (1999), 'Analysis of gene expression in single oocytes and embryos by real-time rapid cycle fluorescence monitored RT-PCR', *Molecular Human Reproduction*, vol. 5, pp. 1034-1039.

Stewart, D.R. and VandeVoort, C.A. (1999), 'Relaxin secretion by human granulosa cell culture is predictive of in-vitro fertilization–embryo transfer success', *Human Reproduction*, vol. 14, pp. 338-344.

Stojanov, T., Alechna, S. and O'Neill, C. (1999), 'In-vitro fertilization and culture of mouse embryos in vitro significantly retards the onset of insulin-like growth factor-II expression from the zygotic genome', *Molecular Human Reproduction*, vol. 5, pp. 116-124.

Surani, M.A. (1999), 'Reprogramming a somatic nucleus by trans-modification activity in germ cells', *Seminars in Cell and Developmental Biology*, vol. 10, pp. 273-277.

Sutovsky, P., Ramalho-Santos, J., Moreno, R.D., Oko, R., Hewitson, L. and Schatten, G. (1999), 'On-stage selection of single round spermatids using a vital, mitochondrion-specific fluorescent probe MitoTrackerTM and high resolution differential interference contrast microscopy', *Human Reproduction*, vol. 14, pp. 2301-2312.

Tesarik, J. and Greco, E. (1999), 'The probability of abnormal preimplantation development can be predicted by a single static observation on pronuclear stage morphology', *Human Reproduction*, vol. 14, pp. 1318-1323.

Turner, K., Martin, K.L., Woodward, B.J., Lenton, E.A. and Leese, H.J. (1994), 'Comparison of pyruvate uptake by embryos derived from conception and non-conception natural cycles', *Human Reproduction*, vol. 9, pp. 2362-2366.

Van Blerkom, J. (1997), 'Can the developmental competence of early human embryos be predicted effectively in the clinical IVF laboratory?', *Human Reproduction*, vol. 12, pp. 1610-1614.

Van Blerkom, J. (1998), 'Epigenetic influences on oocyte developmental competence: perifollicular vascularity and intrafollicular oxygen', *Journal of Assisted Reproduction and Generics*, vol. 15, pp. 226-234.

Van Royen, E., Mangelschots, K., De Neubourg, D., Valkenburg, M., Van de Meerssche, M., Ryckaert, G., Eestermans, W. and Gerris, J. (1999), 'Characterization of a top quality embryo, a step towards single-embryo transfer', *Human Reproduction*, vol. 14, pp. 2345-2349.

Walker, S.K., Hartwich, K.M. and Seamark, R.F. (1996), 'The production of unusually large offspring following embryo manipulation: concepts and challenges', *Theriogenology*, vol. 45, pp. 111-120.

Weber, R.J., Pedersen, R.A., Wianny, F., Evans, M.J. and Zernika-Goetz, M. (1999), 'Polarity of the mouse embryo is anticipated before implantation', *Development*, vol. 126, pp. 5591-5598.

Wilmut, I., Schnieke, A.E., McWhir, A.J. and Campbell, K.H.S. (1997), 'Viable offspring derived from fetal and adult mammalian cells', *Nature*, vol. 385, pp. 810-812.

Winston, N.J., Braude, P.R. and Johnson, M.H (1993), 'Are failed fertilized oocytes useful?', *Human Reproduction*, vol. 8, pp. 503-507.

Ziomek, C.A. and Johnson, M.H. (1981), 'Properties of polar and apolar cells from the 16-cell mouse morula', *Roux's Archives for Developmental Biology*, vol. 190, pp. 287-296.

Part II
ETHICS

5 Overview: Ethical Issues

VERONICA ENGLISH[1] AND INEZ DE BEAUFORT

Introduction

Embryo research has been one of the most hotly debated topics in medical ethics over the last two decades. One of the pioneers of IVF, Professor Bob Edwards, was one of the first people to consider the ethical dilemmas raised by his attempts to fertilize human oocytes outside the body. As early as 1971 Edwards was predicting public unease about work on human embryos and was calling for mechanisms to promote public debate and for some form of public scrutiny of work in this area. Nearly thirty years later the subject is still a matter of fierce debate with little prospect of international agreement.

Pluralism and the status of the embryo

The central point of argument, but by no means the only controversial aspect of the debate on embryo research, is the status of the embryo which has been the subject of radical disagreement on both a descriptive and normative level. A spectrum of views are represented in most societies from those who believe the embryo has the same status as an adult human being to those who perceive the embryo to be no more than a collection of cells. These two polarized views hide a multitude of opinion in between. The middle ground in this debate is adopted by those who believe that, because of its potential to become a person, the embryo deserves some, but not absolute, respect and that this respect must be weighed against the potential benefits of research. (Different perspectives on the status of the embryo and "personhood" are considered in more detail in chapter 8.)

This debate goes to the very heart of our views about life itself, raising complex philosophical questions about when life begins and when people begin to matter morally. Many volumes have been written and, no doubt, will continue to be written on this subject covering ethical, legal,

---

[1] The views expressed in this paper are those of the authors and not those of the British Medical Association.

developmental, cultural and religious perspectives. Factual answers, however, inevitably remain elusive since the question itself is not entirely a factual one but is, in part, a matter of belief. Ethical arguments can be used to justify whatever stage of development we choose to regard as morally relevant - whether when the sperm and egg come together as a single entity, the fusion of the genetic material or the moment of implantation - but there is no single point that clearly emerges from ethical discourse.

This is not only an interesting topic for philosophical debate but it also has practical implications for public policy. The status one chooses to afford to the human embryo will have a direct bearing on what level of protection it should receive. Those who believe that the embryo, from the moment of conception, has the full status of any other human being argue strongly that embryos must be afforded full protection in accordance with that status. Thus, destroying a human embryo is no different, morally, from destroying an existing child or adult. In their view, therefore, all research on human embryos is intrinsically wrong and must be prohibited. The opposite view will be taken by those who see the embryo merely as a collection of cells who will focus, instead, on the potential benefits of the research. It is essential that the rights of citizens who find themselves in the moral minority on either side of the debate must be considered, but how are these conflicting view points to be reconciled? Those who take a conservative position on the status of the embryo will not be content simply to personally refrain from causing harm to embryos but will also insist on absolute prohibitions on embryo research. In a pluralist society, should the views of one group be imposed on others who do not share their beliefs? Tolerance of, and respect for, the viewpoint of others is an important principle but this does not mean that there can be no restrictions on individual action. A state in which every citizen lived by their own moral code, without clearly defined rules, would lack social cohesion and it is difficult to envisage how it could survive without degenerating into lawlessness. So tolerance of different viewpoints does not imply that those viewpoints will always prevail.

Given the range of views represented in the embryo debate, it is interesting to consider whether there is such a thing as a collective national morality which leads countries such as Germany and Austria to prohibit embryo research and those such as the United Kingdom and Sweden to permit it. Without doubt the whole range of opinions will be reflected in the population of each country but perhaps the balance of opinion is influenced by the country in which we live. Our personal views on a whole range of issues are, inevitably, shaped to some extent by factors such as the religious, cultural, legal, constitutional, social and political background of our society. These factors will not only influence the dominant view about the status of the embryo but also the model of regulation, if any, most suited to that society. Recognizing this, it is essential for each country to go through the process of debate and dialogue to enable the citizens of each country to identify the moral position that sits most comfortably with their own beliefs and values. At a time of increasing harmonization throughout Europe this is one area in which the search for a consensus view is likely to be unsuccessful.

Whilst each country can, and does, have its own regulations and prohibitions in relation to embryo research, this does not mean that they are unaffected by the policies of other countries. With increasing integration in Europe and beyond, the views and actions of different countries inevitably impact upon each other. This can lead to tensions and present ethical dilemmas.

Using the results of "unethical" research

Through the international literature, conferences and personal contacts, those working in countries that prohibit embryo research will inevitably be aware of results of research carried out elsewhere. The question this raises is to what extent it is right for them to utilize the results of research that is, in their own country, both illegal and considered to be unethical. Whilst the broader issue of using the results of unethical research has received considerable attention in the literature, most notably in relation to the results of Nazi experiments, the issue here is fundamentally different. This difference is based on a distinction between research that almost everybody considers to be unethical and that which gives rise to genuine moral controversy. The type of research carried out in the Nazi era is considered to be intrinsically unethical and is globally condemned. Embryo research, on the other hand, is permitted and considered ethically acceptable in some countries but prohibited and condemned in others. This issue has received far less attention.

Again, in addition to the interesting ethical debate this gives rise to, there are practical questions that need to be addressed. In view of the fact that some countries prohibit all embryo research, and a higher number prohibit the creation of embryos for research, how does that affect clinical practice in those countries? Where embryo research is used to develop new treatment options, or to improve the efficacy or safety of an existing procedure, professionals offering infertility services in those countries that prohibit embryo research have two options: either they use the information for the benefit of their patients or they do not. Behind this apparently straightforward question lies a complex ethical debate about whether it is right for those countries to benefit from the results of research considered, by their country, to be unethical; this is discussed in chapter 6 and is not addressed here. But, for those who are able to overcome this apparent moral inconsistency there is a need to find pragmatic, workable and safe ways of making new techniques available to patients in those countries.

One option is for those professionals working in countries that prohibit embryo research to follow the literature of developments from the research carried out in other countries and to use that information to modify their own clinical practice. In many ways this is simply an extension of existing practice. It is not necessary for individual clinics to repeat every piece of research in their own laboratory before making any changes to their protocols. Where difficulties could arise, however, is where a new technique has been devised that requires particular skills, training and expertise to be carried out effectively and safely. Intra-cytoplasmic sperm injection (ICSI) and the embryo biopsy required for preimplantation genetic diagnosis (PGD) are examples of such techniques. Where it is not possible to become proficient using research embryos, the techniques may be adopted following a review of the literature without the benefit of practical experience. In these cases, there could be an increased risk of causing damage to the embryo that might be harmful to both the woman and her future child. Those seeking treatment, for whom these techniques offer the best chance of success may, despite the inherent risks and uncertainties, be willing to accept the increased risk. But there are generally limits to the level of risk even competent adults may validly consent to.

If these risks are considered too great, another option is for those patients requiring the treatment to visit another country where the procedure is already established. This form of "reproductive tourism" has been operating for a number of years. It has been particularly evident in the field of reproduction where patients have traveled to other countries to evade restrictive entrance criteria for fertility treatment or to seek treatments not available in their home country. With increasing free trade and transfer of goods and services throughout Europe, medical treatment may become more like any other commodity bought from the best, cheapest, safest or most convenient supplier. Whilst this would protect those patients, by ensuring that those providing the treatment are appropriately trained, there are concerns about the level of service available to those who are either unable or unwilling to travel to another country. Initially the difference in the quality of the service will be small, but over a period of time, the gap between the service and treatments available will grow. If a new procedure becomes the accepted standard treatment option for particular patients - such as ICSI for patients with male factor infertility - genuine questions will arise about the acceptability of those countries that do not offer it, continuing to provide only standard IVF which could, for those patients, be considered substandard treatment.

A third option would be for those working in reproduction, who are not opposed to embryo research, to travel to countries where research is permitted to learn the technique. The individual professional would, personally, be involved in the research but not in the country where it is forbidden. But operator training is only one part of the necessary preparation for introducing new techniques. Safeguards are also needed to ensure that the equipment and facilities in the laboratory, where the treatment is to take place, are suitable. This may require the trainer visiting the country that prohibits research in order to oversee the setting up of the equipment and facilities. It could be argued that a country permitting such close links to the research and so clearly benefiting from its results, is not serious about its moral opposition to the research itself. Leaving aside the moral arguments about the acceptability of the individual and the citizens of the country benefiting from the research it considers to be unethical, however, this pragmatic approach would enable citizens of that country to have safe access to the latest developments in treatment services.

There is thus a moral tension between a country's desire to protect human embryos, by prohibiting their use for research, and its wish to provide the best possible treatments for its citizens. This tension is likely to grow as the range of potential benefits arising from embryo research increases. Until recently, the benefits of embryo research have been restricted to areas associated with reproduction - whether aimed at improving methods of fertility treatment or developing techniques to avoid the birth of children with severe genetic disorders. Whilst important, the potential benefits affect only a small number of people and although they may be life-enhancing they are not, in themselves, life-saving. New areas of embryo research have now been identified which go beyond this limited sphere which not only have the potential to benefit huge numbers of the population of all countries but also have the potential to save lives. The obvious example is recent research on embryonic stem cells aimed at the development of tissue for transplantation (this is addressed in chapter 9). This presents a huge challenge for those countries that prohibit embryo research on moral grounds.

Use of one or a combination of the practical solutions suggested above would mean that a prohibition on embryo research need not hinder the development of IVF services in that country or necessarily restrict the range of treatments available to its citizens. But, by adopting such solutions, the country leaves itself open to claims of moral inconsistency and, arguably, its credibility in promoting the immorality of such research is seriously compromised.

Cloning

A popular theme of both ethical and public debate over the last few years has been human cloning. A wide variety of activities have been included under the general heading of "cloning". Those that involve the creation and use of embryos can be divided into two distinct types based on the ultimate objective. Where the objective is deliberately to create genetically identical individuals, this is often referred to as "reproductive cloning". This technique may, theoretically, be used either to create an individual with the same genetic make-up as an existing individual - by cell nuclear replacement techniques - or to deliberately produce monozygotic twins - either by cell nuclear replacement or embryo splitting - with the primary intention of increasing the number of embryos available for transfer in an IVF cycle. Although the ethical arguments differ, both of these techniques have been prohibited in a broad statement in the Additional Protocol to the Council of Europe's Convention on Human Rights and Biomedicine.

The second category of activities do not involve the creation of genetically identical individuals, but aim to produce an unlimited source of tissue for transplantation. It is proposed that undifferentiated embryonic stem cells, from early embryos, could be stimulated to differentiate into whatever type of tissue was needed - neural tissue for the treatment of degenerative diseases such as Parkinsons disease, bone marrow for leukemia sufferers, islet cells for diabetes, muscle tissue for the repair of a damaged heart or skin for treating burns victims. A further development would be to produce tissue which was immunologically compatible to the recipient. This could be achieved by transferring the nucleus from one of the patient's own somatic cells into an enucleated donor egg which would then be stimulated to begin cell-division but only to the stage needed to separate and culture the embryonic stem cells. This would succeed, not only in overcoming the shortage of tissue for transplantation but also, because the cells would be generated using the patient's own DNA, the tissue would be fully compatible so there would be no need for the use of immunosuppressive drugs. This use of cloning techniques has potentially huge implications for a vast number of people and presents a serious challenge to those who are morally opposed to all embryo research. Issues around cloning are discussed in chapter 9.

Informed consent

The development of any new technique in medical practice involves a continuum from basic research, through innovative therapy (or therapeutic research) to standard clinical practice. Until a procedure reaches the end of this spectrum, and is accepted as standard clinical practice, it must be considered a form of experimentation, subject to rigorous scientific and ethical scrutiny. In any form of experimentation, informed consent is a necessary requirement but is not, in itself, sufficient to justify the research on ethical grounds. With embryo research, it is the donors of the gametes who must give consent to the use of embryos for basic research. As the research moves to the stage where a new procedure is to be used for the first time in clinical practice (the therapeutic research stage) consent is needed both for the use of embryos and for the transfer of the embryos to the uterus for gestation. The provision of accurate information at this stage is crucial, enabling the woman concerned to make an informed decision about whether to proceed on the basis of a clear understanding of the inherent risks and uncertainties. There are, however, questions about the validity of an individual's consent to highly experimental procedures, particularly when it may be perceived as that individual's only, or at the least the best, chance to have a desperately wanted child. There are also limits to the level of risk an individual may validly consent to. This and other issues around consent are explored in chapter 7.

6 Between Pragmatism and Principles?

On the morality of using the results of research that a country considers immoral

INEZ DE BEAUFORT AND VERONICA ENGLISH[1]

Introduction

> *Imagine a country, A, where research on embryos is considered to be immoral and is therefore prohibited by law. Should doctors or patients in country A use the results of research on embryos carried out elsewhere, say in country B, where such research is considered morally acceptable and is legal?*

This chapter discusses some of the arguments in favour of permitting country A to use the results of embryo research undertaken in country B and the counter arguments opposing such use. It does not discuss the moral arguments about the use of embryos for research but, rather, begins from the position that different European countries have opposing moral views on which they have based their laws. Given the diverse nature of laws across Europe on embryo research, we focus on the ethical debate about the extent to which those countries that prohibit embryo research should benefit from the results of that research carried out elsewhere. This is a very real problem that will, in our view, pose itself more often in the future in the European Union.   One can think of the development of new techniques for improving infertility treatment, such as intra cytoplasmic sperm injection (ICSI) and, beyond the scope of fertility treatment, research using embryonic stem cells for the development of tissue for transplantation. Should these procedures be used in countries that consider the research that led to their development to be immoral?

---

[1] The views expressed in this chapter are those of the authors and not those of the British Medical Association.

The following arguments will be considered:

1. Pragmatism versus Consistency
2. Non-complicity versus Complicity
3. Individual Citizen versus Democracy.
4. Best Option versus Safety
5. Reciprocity versus Unfairness

Pragmatism versus consistency

The pragmatic argument

The pragmatic argument is based on the view that it would be impractical not to use the results of the research. Intra cytoplasmic sperm injection (ICSI) was developed as a technique to help couples with male infertility to have a child. In developing the technique, it was necessary to carry out research on embryos created for that purpose and discarded after the research. The research has already been carried out, it is known that the technique is safe and effective and now it is available in clinical practice in country B. Even if country A would not allow the research, it is argued that its citizens should have access to ICSI. Once the information is available, it would be impractical not to use it, the research has been carried out anyway, the results are available and it is better that some good comes of it. If not, the patients who need the treatment would suffer. After all, it is not the resulting techniques that are considered to be immoral; country A does not have any objection to ICSI, only to the research that led to it.

In reality, it is very difficult to isolate that knowledge obtained from research involving embryos from existing knowledge or that obtained from other types of research. Knowledge does not form separate packages of information so that particular bits can be split off and selectively used but rather it develops layer upon layer so that our overall knowledge is gradually increased. Over time information obtained from embryo research interweaves with existing information and becomes part of the "common knowledge" of the community.   Once an individual has a piece of information, it is impossible not to know it. One can hardly suggest that doctors should impose upon themselves a strict form of self-censorship and should not read the literature; or, knowing that a new technique exists should not attempt to provide the best possible treatment for their patients.

The consistency argument

According to the consistency argument it would be inconsistent and hypocritical to forbid the research on the one hand and profit from the research carried out elsewhere on the other. This could also be called the "you can't have your cake and eat it" argument. It is dishonest to oppose embryo research and benefit from the results in the same way that it would be considered dishonest to oppose abortion but to accept a transplant of fetal tissue. Either one takes the view that the research, or the abortion, is unacceptable and faces the consequences - in terms of not benefiting from it - or one decides that the ends are sufficiently important to justify the means. You cannot have it both ways.

If we could all simply wash our hands in innocence in the way suggested by the pragmatists we could justify just about anything. One would always be free to use the results of someone else's immoral acts. Thus there should be no moral objection to the use of drugs tested on poor people in developing countries who did not give their consent or to us benefiting from the sale of cheap goods produced by child labour.

Non-complicity versus complicity

The non-complicity argument

The non-complicity argument runs as follows: it is not always wrong to profit from the acts of someone else that one considers immoral because one can respect that someone else has a different view on the morality of the act. I can, for example, argue that I think that embryos ought not to be used for research, but that living in a pluralist world I have to accept and respect that others have different views. I do not have the right to impose my views on someone else. Although I do not agree with them I still respect their view and therefore I am not an accomplice if I use the results of their research. This argument is different from the pragmatic argument in the sense that it is based on respect for differing moral opinions in a deeper sense than "it happens anyway, so why not use the results". One is not an accomplice because one believes it is highly important that differing views are respected.

How to judge the non-complicity argument depends on one's judgment on the immorality of the acts and whether one accepts that others may have good reasons not to consider those acts immoral. Obviously, the stronger one feels, and the stronger one considers one's arguments to be, the more difficult it is to accept that others do not agree and to respect their views. Therefore, the stronger one's opposition to the use of embryos for research, the more strained the justification for profiting from the results would be. If one is convinced that abortion is tantamount to murder and that the use of embryos is sacrificing potential persons, it is difficult to respect that others do not think it is murder at all and to profit from the results of such terrible acts.

What is interesting about this argument is that it would not hold for all moral views. It would limit the profiting or use to certain categories of act on which moral opinion differs and to those where there is moral room to respect both for the fact that others have different views and possibly to respect the arguments underlying those differing views. Therefore the argument is less susceptible, although not immune, to a slippery slope criticism. It would not hold for example for using the results of research based on torture. The point of view that torture is immoral is one that is universally accepted and one cannot respect the views of those who would argue that torture is acceptable. The non-complicity argument presupposes respect for the views of those with whom one does not agree.

The complicity argument

If one forbids embryo research for moral reasons regarding the moral status of the embryo, one considers certain forms of research to be morally wrong. In using the results of that research one would, in a certain way, become an accomplice in the wrongdoing of someone else. One could argue that in using the results of research one becomes responsible for the immoral acts in two ways. One becomes responsible for what has been done in the past by profiting from it and for what will be done in the future by not giving the researchers a reason to stop and, to the contrary, giving them a reason to continue – they know the results will be used. (Although they do not need that reason to go on, because since they do not think it is immoral they will proceed anyway.)

The reasons for forbidding the research were moral reasons based on the moral status of the embryo. So, one would expect that country A cares, not only about its "own" embryos, but also about the embryos in country B. Although it has no legal power to stop country B carrying out the research, if country A profits from the results it is therefore condoning it. After all, we are talking about positive acts and decisions (to use embryos for research) and not about natural disasters or awful things that happen and that are nobody's decision. Profiting from tragic situations, such as organ transplantation after a natural death or the use of fetal tissue after a spontaneous abortion, is not at all the same thing.

The non-complicity argument is strained in the eyes of many and could be used to justify too much. Certainly those who strongly disapprove of the research on embryos are likely to argue that any use of the research arising from it makes them complicit in the act. They might argue that the non-complicity argument is, in fact, no more than the pragmatic argument dressed up in a pseudo-elegant moral way and that it is difficult to make a clear distinction between the acts that should and should not be respected. Why, for example, draw the line at torture or child labour and accept abortion and research on embryos? There might also be a concern that the tolerance on which the non-complicity argument is based might lead to indifference and then come very close to the pragmatic argument.

Individual citizen versus democracy

The individual citizen argument

This argument is based on the view that individual citizens or health care providers may not agree with their country's policy and therefore feel individually justified in using the results. In doing so, the individual is not breaking the law of his own country, since he is not carrying out the forbidden research. He simply uses information that has been obtained from legitimate research in another country. He will not worry about being an accomplice, because he does not consider that the research is wrong. This can be compared to a citizen from a country where abortion is forbidden seeking an abortion in a country where abortion is legal.

One could argue that that person would be undermining the law of his own country, and in fact his acts might be considered as criticising the country's law without actually breaking it. But so what? That is his democratic right if he is convinced that the policy in his own country is wrong.

The democracy argument

This line of argument states that individual citizens who do not agree with the policy of their own country must realize that they live in a democratic country and therefore ought to abide by the law that was democratically made. The individual citizen should therefore follow not only the letter of the law but also the spirit of it by refraining from using the results. Whilst allowing each citizen's actions to be guided by his own sense of morality sounds fine in principle, in practice it would lead to complete social breakdown. We cannot have a society in which a person who does not agree with the law may simply ignore it. If, however, there is strong pressure to use the results, that implies that the law should be changed because apparently the citizens do not agree with it or, at least, are not prepared to live with the consequences.

Best option versus safety

The best option argument

This argument considers the outcome for the provision of infertility treatment in country A without using the results and argues that this is not an acceptable option. This argument has some similarities to the pragmatic argument but is slightly different. Instead of saying "the research is available so it may as well be used", this position argues that the consequences of not using the research are so great that the better option is to make a small concession to the general principle by using the results of the research.

Without access to the results of research carried out elsewhere there are two likely outcomes: either new techniques will be applied without the appropriate basic research or the fertility service offered will remain static. If new techniques are adopted, without the preliminary research being undertaken, for example by skipping from animal research to therapeutic research without the basic research stage in between, there is a risk that the woman and her future child will be exposed to greater harm than is necessary. Whilst the woman must be informed of the inherent risks and uncertainties and give informed consent, it is generally agreed that there are limits to what even a competent adult may consent to.

The alternative would be to accept that the only improvements that could be made to existing protocols would be those arising from research not involving human embryos. This would mean, for example, that new techniques developed in country B using embryo research, such as ICSI for the treatment of male factor infertility, would not be available to patients in country A. This may be considered unfair to people living in that country but there may also be a long-term effect on the availability of fertility services in that country. As more efficient techniques become available in country B, questions may be raised about the acceptability of country A continuing to provide treatment that was standard a number of years previously which, compared with developments in other countries, would be considered substandard.

Whilst those working in fertility services in country A do not wish to be directly involved with embryo research itself they also accept that they have a responsibility to their patients to provide the best possible treatment. In order to fulfil this responsibility, they may be prepared to soften their own stance slightly to enable them to follow the literature and make use of the information reported. They may see this as a small concession not involving a major shift in their principles.

The safety argument

In addition to the moral inconsistency in the best option argument, there are also practical difficulties. There are serious questions about the acceptability of an individual reading about a new technique in the literature and then simply applying it in clinical practice. Whilst this may be acceptable for minor amendments to the treatment protocol, for the use of newly developed techniques, such as ICSI, that require particular skills and expertise in order to be used safely, it could be argued that this is not a reasonable option. In reality, each person using the technique needs, at the very least, to have the procedure overseen by someone with experience gained from the research. It may be that the individual from country A would also need to demonstrate proficiency with the technique using embryos that are not to be used for treatment, in order to ensure that the procedure itself has not damaged the embryo. This raises difficulties for the best option argument because the minor concession of simply reading the literature would raise serious concerns about safety. In reality, the link between those providing the treatment and those involved with the research would need to be much closer.

Reciprocity versus unfairness

The reciprocity argument

The reciprocity argument acknowledges that individual countries will each have different research priorities and argues that the combined knowledge of this research should be used for the benefit of citizens in the entire European Union. It focuses on the need for co-operation and emphasises that countries should share the results of the research they undertake. Country A may not be carrying out embryo research but it is carrying out other research that may not be possible, or permissible in other parts of Europe. If Country A would not object to the results of its research being used by country B, there should be no objection by country B to country A using its results.

The unfairness argument

This line of argument states that it is unfair for a country to profit from research it condemns because that country has not contributed in any way to that research. An interesting issue is the following: what if a doctor from country A travels to country B in order to carry out embryo research using embryos donated by the citizens of country B. This type of "research tourism" is becoming very common with an increasing international scientific and medical community. If the sole purpose of the exercise is for the doctor to return to country A with the knowledge and experience of new techniques, the citizens of country B could argue that it is unfair that they donate their embryos for research from which the citizens of another country profit. It is not unfair in the sense that the citizens from country B are robbed of benefit, because they have exactly the same advantages and availability of new techniques. The unfairness, however, would lie in the absence of reciprocity, in the fact that others who have not contributed to the research, in fact who have opposed the research, are benefiting from it. This could lead to arguments such as "these were our embryos, the research was done with our tax money and they have done nothing" and "they say that what we do is immoral, condemn us for it, but still profit from the results. That is not only inconsistent, it is also grossly unfair."

Of course, absence of reciprocity is not always a reason to prevent someone from profiting from the accomplishments of someone else. It depends on the reasons why the person (or country) that profits did not contribute to the results. If he could not contribute, because of poverty for example, the situation is very different. Where he did not contribute because he believed the research to be immoral, and in fact condemned those carrying out the research, the unfairness argument holds.

The unfairness argument also includes issues around scarcity. If medical tourism became so popular that large numbers of people from country A were visiting country B for treatment, this could lead to a scarcity in the services available in country B. This could lead to citizens of country B not being treated, or being treated less or later; this would be unfair in a different way. They would be robbed of the personal benefits accruing to them of the research carried out in their country. This could be construed either as an argument to provide the treatment in country A or to argue that, unfortunately, the treatment cannot be made available for the citizens of country A for reasons of fairness.

Conclusions

In our view, the arguments against country A using the results of research carried out in country B are more persuasive than those in favour of such use. We are inclined, therefore, to support the "you can't have your cake and eat it" line of argument. The practical implication of adopting this position is that country A needs to choose either:

1.   that it feels very strongly about protecting embryos and therefore ought not to use the research result; or
2.   that it wants to use the results and therefore should reconsider its law.

What holds for a country as a whole (stick to the law and face the consequences or change it), however, is different from the choices of individual citizens. Those who do not agree with the moral stance of their country will not be inconsistent or hypocritical if they use the results. But consideration needs to be given to the practical strategies that could be adopted for ensuring safe and effective use of new techniques. The argument from respect for differing views is an interesting one that ought to be developed further in this context.

Our final conclusion is that the problem we have addressed has not received much attention in the moral debate on research on embryos although it is a highly relevant problem in the European Union, particularly in the light of the European Convention on Human Rights and Biomedicine. The desire and pressure to use the results of embryo research is likely to grow as the potential benefits arising from it increase. If it proves possible to use human embryonic stem cells to develop various types of tissue for transplantation, for example, the benefit to citizens in all countries would be huge. If such potentially life-saving options arise, this presents a serious challenge to those countries who must decide whether to make use of the development despite their moral opposition to the research that made it possible, or to stick to their principles and forgo the benefits. The debate has focussed, so far, on differing views on the status of the embryo. An equally important, and pressing question is: if we agree that we do not agree on the morality of research on embryos what are the consequences?

7 Information Disclosure and Consent

SHEILA A.M. MCLEAN

It is now widely accepted that, for any clinical intervention to be valid in ethics or in law, there must be a pre-existing free and voluntary consent to participation from the individual concerned.[1] Although definitions of consent, and in particular the amount of information required to make a consent 'informed'[2], vary from jurisdiction to jurisdiction, the principle that consent is an essential trigger of lawful and ethical intervention remains resolutely in place as an unavoidable precursor of a 'good' and lawful medical act.

That said, it is by no means a simple task to unpick from the rhetoric of patient autonomy and self-determination what in fact characterises or describes a valid and meaningful consent. In part, this is arguably because of the concentration on the outcome (that is the consent) itself rather than on the process by which a meaningful consent is obtained.[3] The validity of a consent, and the concomitant authority to intervene in the clinical setting, will to an extent hinge on two critical factors: first, the nature of the procedure and second the quality and extent of information provided (arguably including the circumstances in which provision of information is made). This chapter will briefly address each of these issues in turn.

The nature of the intervention

It is worth at this stage noting that clinical interventions can broadly be described for convenience as either 'standard' or 'experimental'. In the 'standard' or ordinary medical intervention, the requirement in the United Kingdom (and in many other countries) is essentially that 'material' risks must be disclosed before a person is properly informed.[4] In addition, it is generally agreed that alternatives should be canvassed, and it is, of course, expected that the benefits of a treatment will also be explored. The last of these requirements is seldom, if ever, controversial, but the first two may be. However, even in routine medical interventions, it is by no means clear

67

what information needs to be disclosed before an individual can be said to have given a legally valid consent. Arguments range from the insistence that all information in the doctor's possession must be disclosed,[5] to a more professional standard which would endorse leaving decisions about the extent of necessary disclosure substantially to clinicians.[6]

In situations which are described as 'experimental', however, the standard of disclosure required is generally conceded to be more demanding and perhaps better defined.   This was clearly stated in the Canadian case of *Halushka* v *University of Saskatchewan*.[7] In this case, the court made a clear statement on the quality of dialogue required to satisfy the disclosure requirements in experimental procedures, saying:

> The duty imposed on those who engage in medical research....to those who offer themselves as subjects for experimentation...is at least as great as, if not greater than the duty owed by the ordinary physician or surgeon to his patient. There can be no exceptions to the ordinary requirements of disclosure in the case of research as there may well be in ordinary medical practice....The subject of medical experimentation is entitled to a full and frank disclosure of all the facts, probabilities and options which a reasonable man might be expected to consider before giving his consent.[8]

This commitment to full disclosure is also recognised in international documents such as the Declaration of Helsinki (as amended), the guidance to which research protocols are expected to adhere, as well as being absorbed into the laws of many jurisdictions.   This is significant for assisted conception, as some of its manifestations may be described more readily as experiments than as 'standard' medical practice.   Of course, for some - such as Corea[9]- assisted conception is in its entirety evidence of a massive experiment on (usually) women.   This is, however, as much a cultural as a clinical assertion.   In terms of the clinical, it could, of course, be argued that some kinds of assisted reproduction have now been in use for so long that their categorisation as medical rather than social experiments would be unreasonable.

However, even if this were the case, the techniques of assisted conception continue to develop and it is here that caution is required in terms of categorisation, with the consequential impact on information disclosure.   Techniques like preimplantation genetic diagnosis (PGD) for example, cannot claim to hold a place in standard medical treatment, yet PGD is seen by some as being legitimately offered as part of IVF.   Even if we assume that IVF has crossed the line between experiment and standard, not an unarguable assumption, the availability of PGD is a classic example of the complexity of decision making, which renders a simple acquiescence to assisted conception problematic ethically and legally.   In other words, even if disclosure standards are met in the agreement to participate in IVF, that is for the basic intervention, the question remains whether or not each consequence of that intervention must also be canvassed before the consent is real.   Thus, from being an apparently monolithic exercise, arguably each step of the technique, each nuance of its consequences, should be divulged before a purported consent can truly be real and ethically and legally valid. Indeed, this might remain the case even if the techniques associated with a non-experimental intervention are themselves able to be categorised as 'standard'.

As has been said, experimental procedures demand a higher level of information disclosure in order to enhance the capacity of the individual to maximise autonomy and make a choice which is meaningful to him or her self.   Continuing with the example of PGD, this would therefore require that information is disclosed about what is *not* known as well as what *is* known.   For example, it would be necessary to explain whether or not embryos found to be genetically compromised will be destroyed, and whether or not there is any evidence that PGD itself poses risks to the embryo.   In addition, the individual who is invited to accede to procedures such as PGD should be aware that any information which is disclosed may be based on a relative shortfall of available information, given the relative infrequency of its use to date.   In their joint consultation document[10], for example, the Human Fertilisation and Embryology Authority and the Advisory Committee on Genetic Testing note that only "[f]our centres in the UK are currently licensed to carry out PGD and one centre for the embryo biopsy part of the procedure only".[11]   Moreover, individuals should also - in line with the strict legal position - be informed that the procedure is, in itself, new and relatively untested.   Information should also, arguably, include any potential harm to the potential child, thus attenuating the usual notion of consent from the individual on whom the procedure is to be carried out to the risks which might arise for the child.

Although it has been suggested that a line can be drawn between standard and experimental procedures, it is, unfortunately, increasingly common to blur the line between them.   One clear example of this, which has resonance in the area of assisted reproduction also, is the case of gene 'therapy'.   As Churchill *et al*, have said, '[t]he habitual tendency in clinical research settings to conflate research and therapy is especially evident in the current usage of the term gene therapy'.[12] The rationale for this is not difficult to find.   Orkin and Motulsky state that:

Expectations of current gene therapy have been over-sold.   Overzealous representation of clinical gene therapy has obscured the exploratory nature of the initial studies, colored the manner in which findings are portrayed to the scientific press and public, and led to the widely held, but mistaken, perception that clinical gene therapy is already highly successful.[13]

Thus, if a technique is described in therapeutic rather than experimental terms, it may lead to assumptions about its value and its likely success, quite apart from the reduced stringency - in terms of disclosure - which would be required by the law.

It can be concluded, therefore, that acceptance of the fundamental (even non-experimental) intervention required by assisted conception cannot be presumed, legally or ethically, to imply an agreement to everything that follows. Although it could be argued that this is also the case in what has been referred to as the standard medical act, the need to make this assertion is even more obvious in these situations. Yet, as the concommitant techniques of assisted conception gain scientific acceptance, the temptation not to assume the additional disclosure burden is real. For example, it is now common practice to freeze gametes and embryos as a direct consequence of the methods of IVF, yet little systematic evidence has been gathered about the harm that may be caused to the gametes or embryos as a result. More topically, the recent struggle in the UK for women to be permitted to use frozen ova - taken and stored in advance of treatment which was likely to render the women infertile - challenged the Human Fertilisation and Embryology Authority (HFEA) essentially to conclude on what was science fact and what was science speculation.

Having originally refused to permit the use of these ova on the basis of uncertainty about the associated risks, the HFEA ultimately agreed to reverse this decision. The Chairman of the HFEA, Ruth Deech, is quoted as having said:

> We can only make our decisions based on firm medical evidence. We are pleased that we now have that evidence giving hope to those women who could otherwise have been made infertile.[14]

Freezing of eggs is a relatively new phenomenon whose consequences are as yet relatively poorly understood, yet the demand, for example from cancer patients, for the release of frozen eggs is increasing. As the technology to store eggs improves, so too will the number of women (especially young women) facing possibility of infertility as a result of cancer treatment, seeking to freeze and then subsequently use, their own ova. What is critical is that the agreement of the HFEA is not taken as presupposing that this remains anything other than experimental, and - that being the case - subject to stringent consent requirements. Indeed, it is comforting to note that the author of an independent report also made it clear that risks should be disclosed fully.[15]

What information should be disclosed?

As has been noted, in routine medical interventions, it is expected that risks which are 'material' should be disclosed. This apparently simple assertion, however, disguises real debate over what is, in fact, material. Broadly speaking, the test for materiality can be assessed in one of three distinct ways. First, materiality might be taken to refer to what is material to a specific patient. This is, however, an approach rarely taken in law. The closest we have come to adopting this perspective on disclosure can probably be found in the Australian case of *Rogers* v *Whitaker*[16] in which Gaudron, J. said:

> A patient may have special needs or concerns which, if known to the doctor, will indicate that special or additional information is required. In a case of that kind, the information to be provided will depend on the individual patient concerned.[17]

A more common approach, in the United States at least, is to adopt the 'prudent patient' test - derived from the case of *Canterbury* v *Spence*.[18] The judgement in this case, which - it must be said - is not followed in all US states, requires that information which the 'prudent patient' would wish must be disclosed. This approach has also been followed by the Canadian case of *Reibl* v *Hughes*,[19] but was dismissed - with the exception of Lord Scarman's judgement - in the UK case of *Sidaway* v *Board of Governors of the Bethlem Royal Hospital and the Maudsley Hospital*.[20] The 'prudent patient' test requires the doctor to have regard to facts which it might reasonably be assumed the average or 'prudent' patient might consider to be relevant in reaching a decision on whether or not to accept treatment, subject always to the notion of 'therapeutic privilege'.[21]

In the United Kingdom, however, the test used is that of the 'reasonable doctor'. Decisions, therefore about what information should be disclosed are essentially transferred to clinicians, subject only to the caveat that courts may still hold these decisions to have been negligent. In the (in)famous case of *Bolam* v *Friern Hospital Management Committee*[22] the court made it clear that a doctor will not be negligent if he or she acts in accordance with a practice accepted as reasonable by a responsible body of medical opinion. Although it was first thought by some commentators that this test would only apply in operational matters and might not extend to issues of information disclosure, this hope was dashed by the case of *Gold* v *Haringey Health Authority*[23] and a number of subsequent judgements.

Assisted conception

Whether or not assisted conception can either generally or in part be described as experimental, it presents one further hurdle to the obtaining of a genuinely valid consent.   The situation in which the infertile find themselves may lead many to be prepared to assume enormous physical and emotional risks, in order to satisfy their desire to reproduce.   Indeed, the very platform upon which assisted reproduction practitioners justify their practice - that it meets the needs of often desperate people - might be used as an argument to question, rather than to assert, the validity of their agreement to participate. In other words, the anxiety and distress that generally accompany infertility - at least for those who choose to opt for assisted conception rather than childlessness - might be though to place an increased onus on the clinician, to ensure both that the techniques on offer are thoroughly based in scientific experience and that the process of information disclosure transcends the somewhat relaxed requirements of standard medical intervention.

Conclusion

Information disclosure is designed to facilitate - perhaps even enhance - the autonomy of the individual.   As Mason and McCall Smith put it:

> Looked at from the ethical point of view, the matter is one of self-determination. A person should not be exposed to a risk of damage unless he has agreed to that risk and he cannot properly agree to - or, equally importantly, make a choice between - risks, in the absence of factual information.[24]

Protecting doctors from subsequent litigation is a secondary function. However, it must be asked whether or not the full panoply of the physical and psychological consequences of, for example, ovarian hyperstimulation, receipt of donated gametes, and so on are either fully known and explained or fully explicable.   If known, but not explained, then - in the UK at least - the doctor's failure to make disclosure would be judged against the practice of his or her peers.   This test, which seems weak to many at the best of times, is particularly ill-suited to the event that is assisted reproduction.

Arguably, in fact, the only test which could satisfy the needs of those involved in this enterprise is that which concentrates solely on the individual patient. The pressures and anxieties of infertility, coupled with the consequences of attempting to circumvent it, seem to argue for the highest possible level of disclosure tailored to that particular individual. As the clinician involved will require to know the patient perhaps better than in many other medical interventions, the practical impediments to tailoring information at the individual rather than the objective level disappear.

So far as what is known is concerned, it is of course arguable that people are free to act on lack of information should they so choose. However, this is only an autonomous act when they are aware that information is *not* known and agree to take that risk.

Three purposes are served by accepting that medical advance exposes more people to 'treatments' which are essentially experimental and for which the value of a real consent cannot be underestimated. First, and of paramount importance, the provision of adequate and honest information protects the individual from the unwarranted or uninformed assumption of authority over their bodies. The mere availability of additional 'choice' - such as is apparently offered by assisted conception - is not sufficient to guarantee that an individual's apparent consent is sufficient to meet what should be, it has been argued, stringent standards. The critical issue is that '...a real choice demands an element of control. Control, albeit not necessarily in terms of the technical, is predicated on the availability of information and the power to contribute to the ways in which services are offered an organised'.[25] Although few choices can be said to be truly free of pressure, or even based on every available piece of information, reproductive choice is of such significance to individuals that every effort must be made to ensure that they are empowered. If this means unpicking the procedures and providing information about all aspects of the intervention, describing clearly what is experimental and what is not, then so be it.

Second, the welfare of any future children can also be taken into consideration - both an ethical and a legal requirement.[26] And third, appropriate dialogue, properly recorded, can protect the provider of the services from subsequent challenge or litigation. Ultimately, the complexities of the variety of decisions which require to be made even in the most technologically simple forms of assisted conception require attention to each of the issues raised above *at every stage of the process*.

Notes

1   Most famously, the genesis of this rule is expressed by Cardozo, J., in the case of *Schloendorff* v *Society of New York Hospital* 105 NE 92: 'Every human being of adult years and sound mind has a right to determine what shall be done with his own body...'.

2   It should be noted that the term 'informed consent' when used in its technical sense does not apply in UK law. However, as has been pointed out, it is used de facto if not de jure: Mason, J.K. and McCall Smith, R.A., *Law and Medical Ethics*, 5th Ed., London, Butterworths, 1999, at pp 287-288.

3   For further discussion see Mason and McCall Smith, note 2, *supra*, chapter 10; see also McLean, S.A.M., *A Patient's Right to Know: Information Disclosure, the Doctor and the Law*, Aldershot, Gower, 1989.

4   *Chatterton* v *Gerson* [1981] 1 All ER 257.

5   *Blyth* v *Bloomsbury Health Authority* [1993] 4 Med LR 151.

6   *Sidaway* v *Board of Governors of the Bethlem Royal Hospital and the Maudsley Hospital* [1985] 1 All ER 643.

7   (1965) 53 DLR (2d) 436.

8   at pp 616-7.

9   Corea, G., *The Mother Machine: Reproductive Technologies From Artificial Insemination to Artificial Womb*, London, The Women's Press, 1988.

10   available at http://www.doh.gov.uk/genetics/acgt.htm

11   *ibid*, para 11.

12   Churchill, L.R., *et al*, 'Genetic Research as Therapy: Implications of "Gene Therapy" for Informed Consent', *The Journal of Law, Medicine and Ethics*, 26 (1998):   38, at p. 43

13   Orkin, S.H. and Motulsky, A.G., National Institutes of Health Ad Hoc Committee Report, *Report and Recommendations of the Panel to Assess the N.I.H. Investment in Research on Gene Therapy* (Dec 7, 1995) http://www.nih.gov/od/orda/panelrep.html

14   see wysiwyg://39/http://www.pofsupport.org/info26.htm

15   *id.*

16   BMLR 148 (High Court of Australia, 1992).

17   at p. 159.

18   (1972) 464 F 2d 772.

19   (1980) 114 DLR (3d) 1.

20   note 6, *supra.*

21   This provides the doctor with an explanation for not disclosing information where he or she reasonably believes that disclosure would be detrimental to the health of the patient.

22   [1957] 2 All ER 118.

23   [1987] 2 All ER 888.

24   note 2, *supra*, at p. 278.

25   McLean, S.A.M., *Old Law, New Medicine*, London, Pandora/Rivers Oram, 1999, at p. 31.

26   Human Fertilisation and Embryology Act 1990 s.13(5).

8 The Influence of Pluralism in the Perception of the Status of the Embryo

MAURIZIO MORI

Introduction

By "embryo" I mean the "process of human life from conception to about eight weeks afterwards", and by "pluralism" I mean "ethical pluralism", i.e. a deep and widespread diversity of opinions on ethical matters so that the various moral views are incommensurable because they depend on irreconcilable principles. It is important to keep in mind that this sense of "pluralism" differs from "philosophical pluralism", which is opposed to "philosophical monism", i.e., the view according to which there is only one substance (and reality is at the end "unique"). My topic is about the relationships between the two issues (embryo and ethical pluralism), and I have to clarify how and why the spread of ethical pluralism in contemporary western societies is going to change our perception of the human embryo.

Two preliminary remarks are in order before I try to carry out the task assigned to me. First of all, in the following pages I refer only to the situation in the Western cultures, namely of West Europe, North America and possibly Australia. I have to declare my deep ignorance concerning other cultures, and I disregard them in this presentation. Secondly, I shall look at the issue historically because I think that this approach allows us to find out the real source of controversy and which are the conflicting principles at stake. My thesis is that contemporary emphasis on the status of the embryo is a disguised way of hiding a deeper problem concerning different principles which I hope to identify more clearly.

In Western societies it is important to have a given "status" because a status is generally connected to a *normative* stand, i.e. the ascription of certain duties and rights. In the case of the "human embryo", it is very controversial to ascribe a *status* because of radical disagreements both on the *descriptive* level of analysis as well as on the *normative* one. People disagree both on what the embryo *is* (and therefore on how they perceive it) and also on what protection the embryo should deserve. Some hold that embryos should have rights as any other person and that current situation is a clear violation of basic human rights; while others argue that such a proposal is a mere nonsense, and that embryos are neither persons nor deserve to be treated as if they were persons.

Controversy over the embryo appears to be irreconcilable and many think that it is hopeless to argue on the issue. However, I think that a glance at the history of the subject may provide us a useful path to consider the issue in a new light. I am not too optimistic, since I am well aware of radical disagreement, but I think that my approach can open new perspectives worthwhile to be explored. In this chapter I want to offer an outline of a more general project to be pursued in the future.

The human embryo in the ethical context

My starting point is the following factual observation: when we approach the issue, we cannot forget - even if we usually do - that only a few decades ago the commonsense view and perception of the whole problem was completely different from that of today, and that in a very short time the frame of discussion has changed radically. As a matter of fact, on the *descriptive* level, in the first part of our century it was a commonplace to have a threefold distinction of pre-natal life. So, for instance, the physician and Jesuit Austin O'Malley opens Chapter 3 of his book *The Ethics of Medical Homicide* (1921) remarking without ado that:

> By embryologists from the moment the spermatozoon joins the nucleus of the ovum until the end of the second week of gestation the product of conception is called the *Ovum*; from the end of the second week to the end of the fourth week it is the *Embryo*; from the end of the fourth week to birth it is the *Fetus* (p. 33).

This type of division was used by C.S. Minot in his classic textbook *Human Embryology* (1897) and accepted by L. B. Arey in the second edition of his *Developmental Anatomy* (1930) – while in the first edition (1924) he had a twofold distinction (embryo and fetus). Also the Italian embryologist Giulio Chiarugi holds this threefold distinction in his four volume treatise on embryology (1928-1940), observing that at the beginning there is a "germ" (*germe*), then and "embryo" (*embrione*), and finally a "fetus" (*feto*). This monumental treatise was never reprinted, but Chiarugi also wrote a well-known and successful textbook of human anatomy which had about twenty editions. Starting from the early 1950s Chiarugi gave up his former view to state a twofold distinction (*embrione* and *feto*), even if he never makes clear which (conceptual and empircial) reasons supported his new position or forced him to change his mind. It would be interesting to study why immediately after the Second World War many scholars changed their opinion and accepted the twofold distinction.

Leaving this task to someone else, my thesis is that it was neither decisive scientific discovery nor empirical data that influenced such a change but, more importantly, another sort of change occurred at the *normative* level. Starting from the early 1930s, for the first time in human history, a new attitude emerged in the western culture concerning human control of reproduction. My thesis is that this momentous transformation of the *ethos* had a powerful influence at the *descriptive* level, so that when the new movement started to be visible it influenced embryologists, and when later on in the early 1970s it became prominte, there was a reaction in part of society (the so-called "pro-lifers").

In order to look at this process, it is better to start from scratch and outline the whole story. Some argue that a change concerning human control of procreation started earlier, already in the 19th century. This may be true if we consider people's practical behavior, but we have to acknowledge that only in our century was such behavior openly supported and defended on theoretical grounds. This is what is new in the matter. Looking at religious thinking as evidence of a wider *ethos*, we have to realize that only in 1930 did the Anglican church admit contraception. Before then, according to all christianity any interference in the reproductive process was *absolutely* forbidden. From this point of view, I think that the Roman Catholic position is interesting because it gives an articulated and thoughtful voice to commonsensical views concerning sexuality and reproduction.

In this sense, it is interesting to remark that exactly the same arguments that nowadays are moved against the waste or destruction of embryos, not long ago were used against contraception. Here I give only one quotation: in 1929 the French scholar Pierre Méline wrote that use devices to prevent conception of children is, according to St. Augustine,

"a shameful and unlawful thing"; those who are guilty of it are not really married people, but are falsely using an honorable name "as a veil" for their turpitude. "This is a crime", says Tertullian, "more execrable in a married woman than in a prostitute, for coniugal honour consists of chastity in the act of procreation and of fidelity in the fulfilment of the carnal duty"; and besides, the *prevention of birth is homicidal, for "he who is about to become a man is one already, and all the fruit is contained in the seed".* [1]

I have emphasized the last sentence because it shows that even contraception is clearly considered a form of *homicide*. As evidence of this fact I can say that the same quotation from Tertullian is now usually used in reference to abortion, confirming that from a moral point of view any distinction between pre-conception and post-conception was mostly irrelevant.

In the same perspective, the Jesuit John Ford in 1966 boldly defended the traditional view at the pontifical birth control commission recalling Michelangelo's Creation of Man on the celing of the Sistine Chapel:

> ...God stretching out his finger to touch the finger of Adam and transmit new life to him. This is the moment we are talking about—the *fieri* of a new life. This is the moment of conception. .... contraception (that is contra-ception) involves a will which is turned against new life in this moment. It is against this life, in advance, that is, against its coming to be, its *fieri*. Your conception is your very origin, your link to the community of living persons before you, the first of all gifts received from your parents, your first relationship with God as he stretched out his finger to touch you. In my opinion, there are different ways of expressing the underlying substantial truth: like life itself, the inception of life belongs to God. To attack it is to attack a fundamental human good, to intrude on God's domain. This is why the will to contracept, though essentially different morally from the will to abort, is nevertheless similar to it. And it is noteworthy that among the Catholic theologians who defend contraception today, there are already some who defend therapeutic abortion in certain difficult cases .[2]

These words seem now a bit outmoded or obsolete, but I think that they represent an *ethos* which was deeply rooted in Western culture until the first decades of 20th century, and waned slowly starting from late 1920s up to the early 1970s (being of course still alive and influential in certain social groups). Such remarks show that until that period the real *watershed* concerning the "beginning of *human life*" was sexual intercourse, not conception (in the sense of union of gametes). As a matter of fact, "conception" has at least three different meanings: as the etymology shows, *conceptio* comes from *cum – capere*, i.e. "put together" or "to unite", so that it is an open question to state what are the subjects (or entities) that are to be "put together". They might be the gametes in a woman's body (sexual intercourse), or the union of the gametes themeselves (conception), or the union of the embryo on a woman's womb (nidation). In the past the three different stages were not distinguished, so that *conceptio* meant the beginning of such a process. Furthermore, the whole reproductive process was protected by an *absolute* prohibition from interfering with natural teleology, so that no further question could arise.

It is true that the story concerning the nature of the fetus is rather long, and goes back to Aristotle. But in the past it had only a speculative and abstract character. Even controversies on the time of animation had a purely intellectual interest, since any normative solution was already cleared by the absolute prohibition of any interference with procreative process. This aspect was protected by marriage, which was the *sacramentum magnum* (the great sacrament) because it had to rule all these matters concerning the beginning of life. Discussions on the nature of the fetus were relevant for the issue of a person's responsibility and punishment: but it was clear and granted that both contraception and abortion at any stage were gravely wrong, even if abortion at a later stage was worse than at an earlier one. However, the problem was not about whether one was permissible and the other not, but only about different punishment of two prohibited acts.

After the Second World War this situation started to change significantly, and in the late 1960s the traditional view was reversed: contraception became safer and less cumbersome as well as widely accepted among people as a consequence of what is sometimes called "the sexual revolution", i.e. a deep change of values concerning sexual life. Moreover, the "pill" was decisive because it was conceived as a "drug" and this fact helped to change physicians' negative attitudes towards contraception. Broadly speaking, before the advent of contraception, it was clear that sexuality was primarily *for reproduction*, and that, in a sense, "population concerns" had priority over individuals' desires and wants. Moreover, it was evident that people had no direct *control* over procreation, but could possibly *regulate* it following the nature of the reproductive process (and not interfering with it). Nowdays contraception is so widely accepted that we are led to forget the great "cultural shock" that its public defence engendered at the beginning: for instance an intelligent scholar such as Walter Lippman wrote in 1929 that the Christian churches, and especially the Roman Catholic church, were right in opposing contraception "on principle", and "in recognizing that whether or not birth control is eugenic, hygienic, and economic, *it is the most revolutionary practice in the history of sexual morals*".[3]

There are at least two reasons, I think, to hold such a *revolutionary view* of contraception. On the one hand, if *absolute* prohibition of contraception is abandoned, then the whole idea of having "moral absolutes" is immediately given up: there are no absolute prohibitions any longer. On the other hand, if contraception is permitted, then people are allowed to *control* reproduction and procreative process. If contraception is prohibited, then people can *regulate* the number of offspring "following nature" and have to adjust human choice to such a (natural) norm, while if contraception is morally permitted, then people have the right to directly *control* the reproductive process and the number of their offspring according to human choice (without the bounds of "natural" restraints).

However, in the span of a few decades, a new spirit of the time in favor of contraception overturned the traditional perspective grounded on "natural process". My view is that this point is the real source of our new concern for the "embryo". In this perspective, the "embryo issue" is a sort of *Maginot line* to defend the traditional values of sanctity of life. Since the first defence (absolute prohibition of interferring with procreative process) was already brushed away by the new frame of mind and "contraceptive mentality", the move was to retreat into the citadel of the "embryo", claiming a sort of "absolute respect" at least for such an entity. The easiest move for reaching such a goal is to claim that from the time of conception embryos are to be considered as persons: since in western society human persons deserve a sort of *absolute respect*, this seems enough to guarantee a safe protection of the embryo and the embryo's right to life.

However, this move has its costs, and at the end it appears to be self-defeating. This is clear when we realize that traditionally the prohibition of abortion (as well as of contraception's) is *absolute* while the right to life is not and cannot be of that sort. As a matter of fact it admits at least one exception: self defence. Here we reach a crucial issue which reveals a sort of contradiction hidden in the new defence of the "right to life" of the embryo and helps to individuate the real (moral) principles ruling our case. In order to do it, we can start from a statement of the Congregation for the Doctrine of the Faith claiming that there are two fundamental values connected with the techniques of artificial procreation: "the life of the human being called into existence and the special nature of the transmission of human life in marriage". [4]   As we can see, the "right to life" of the embryo comes first, and the principle concerning "respect for procreation" is following. However, the duty involved in the "right to life" (do not kill!) admits exceptions. Pope John II expressly states that there is "*a true right to self-defence* ... legitimate defence can be not only a right but a grave duty for someone responsible for another's life". [5]   From this premise it follows that abortion would be permitted at least in order to save a woman's life. But, on the other hand, the Congregation forbids "any kind of procured abortion" (I. 1), and therefore consistency requires that abortion is not a violation of the "right to life" but of the principle concerning "the special nature of the transmission of human life in marriage".

This fact explains also why, for the Roman Catholic church, all the further distinctions which are drawn in this matter are irrelevant. For instance, some pro-lifers do admit that contraception is morally licit, but reject any violation of the embryo following conception. However, they would have to clarify the concept of "conception". Some problems have already been hinted at, and new ones are emerging if we consider a passage of the quoted Instruction *Donum Vitae* (1987) of the Congregation for the Doctrine of the Faith: the first official edition (1987) of this document was in Italian and in this version the definition of "zygote" was the following: "The zygote is the cell produced when the *nuclei of the two* gametes have fused". However, in the latin (official) text which was published later (at the beginning of 1988) the definition deletes the emphazied words, making clear that the Congregation does not want enter into "biological matters". Once more, this is further evidence that the real issue is not about the embryo's "right to life", but that the controversy is about the principle concerning the "special nature of the transmission of human life in marriage". This is what is really at stake when we consider the influence of pluralism concerning the perception of the status of the embryo.

Conclusion

If my analysis is right, then in a pluralistic society perception of the human embryo does not depend on different stands concerning the "right to life", but on different perspectives concerning the principle regarding "the special nature of the transmission of human life in marriage". Those who admit contraception and human control of procreation will perceive the embryo simply as a stage of the reproductive process which can be controlled as any former one. In this sense, experimentation on embryo can be permitted and even favored, in as far as it promises beneficial effects for humankind. On the other hand, those who reject contraception and defend the "sanctity of life" and the "transmission of human life in marriage" will see such a will of control as a violation of "nature". My only claim in this chapter was to show that the so-called issue of the "right to life" (or of the "status of the embryo") is irrelevant to the controversy. The real issue at stake is not whether the embryo has an alleged "right to life" from conception, but whether there is or is not an absolute prohibition to interferring and controlling human reproduction. It is at this point that the issue of ethical pluralism becomes relevant. My view is that we have to respect different perspectives, but certainly we should allow each one to pursue his own perspective. Those who believe that there are absolutes are allowed to behave accordingly, but they cannot impose their view on people who think that there are no absolutes. This is the only way to face the issue of the status of the embryo in a pluralistic society.

Notes

1   Méline, Pierre, (1929) *The Moral Law of the Family*, translated by P. Brown, Sands & Co., London, p. 111.

2   Kaiser, Robert Blair,(1987) *The Encyclical that Never Was. The Story of the Pontifical Commission on Population, Family and Birth, 1964-66*,   Sheed & Ward,   London, pp. 209-210.

3   Lippmann, Walter, (1965) *A preface to Morals* (1929) with a new preface by Sidney Hook, Time Incorporated, New York, p. 272 my emphasis.

4   (*Instruction on respect for human Life in Its Origin and on the Dignity of Procreation*, no. 4).

5   John Paul II, *The Gospel of Life. Evangelium Vitae. On the Value and Inviolability of Human Life*, United States Catholic Conference, Publication No. 317-7, Washington, D.C., (text and format from the Libreria Editrice Vaticana, Vatican city), 1995, no. 55.

9 Human Cloning: The Case of the (Preimplantation) Embryo, an Ethical Exploration

GUIDO DE WERT

Introduction

Since the birth of Dolly, the prospect of human cloning has re-emerged as a frontier biomedical issue.[1] Clearly, human cloning raises complex ethical questions. It is important to be aware that there are different sorts of human cloning. At least two distinctions are morally relevant, namely between reproductive cloning and non-reproductive cloning, and between the cloning of adults/children and the cloning of preimplantation embryos (when I use the term embryo, I mean the early, preimplantation embryo). In view of these distinctions, there are at least four categories of human cloning:[2]

- reproductive cloning of adults/children;
- non-reproductive cloning of adults/children, including so-called 'therapeutic' cloning, i.e. cloning for transplantation purposes;[3]
- reproductive embryo cloning;
- non-reproductive embryo cloning.

This ethical exploration concentrates on the reproductive cloning of embryos (REC) and on 'therapeutic' cloning (TC).

What are we talking about?

Let me first very briefly give some background information about the scientific and practical aspects of REC and TC.

Reproductive embryo cloning

Two methods may be used for REC: embryo splitting, more precisely, blastomere separation, and cell nucleus transfer.

REC might serve various purposes in different contexts. *Firstly*, the context of regular IVF. When there is only one embryo available, REC could increase the number of embryos for transfer in a single cycle, thereby increasing the 'take home baby rate' (THBR). Furthermore, for couples who produce only enough embryos for one transfer, REC might provide additional embryos for a subsequent transfer, without having to go through another oocyte retrieval cycle. This strategy could lessen the burdens and costs of IVF.

Some experts seriously doubt whether 'blastomere separation' would increase the odds of women becoming pregnant.[4] They argue, for instance, that genetic heterogeneity (meaning that each embryo is genetically unique) may well be the key to improved pregnancy rates with several embryos transferred. So it would be unlikely that the genetic homogeneity inherent in cloning would improve the THBR. Furthermore, there is substantial evidence that when there are very limited numbers of embryos, the quality of these embryos is also decreased - REC may well only multiply the failure. Other experts, however, are less sceptical.[5] Furthermore, cell nucleus transfer may be an attractive, more efficient, alternative method for REC in the future.[6] One may safely conclude that whether REC will be clinically feasible and valuable for regular IVF practice cannot be determined without further research.

Secondly: in the context of preimplantation genetic diagnosis (PGD), REC may be particularly valuable when there is just one single 'healthy' embryo available for transfer.[7] Again, the aim of REC would be to increase the THBR of medically assisted reproduction.

Thirdly, the context of genetic embryo therapy, an interesting case would be nuclear transplantation in order to prevent mitochondrial disorders.[8] The mitochondria are a kind of power generator in the cell. Each mitochondrion has a small amount of DNA, the so-called mitochondrial DNA (mtDNA). All the mitochondria in an egg that has come from the mother so that genetic defects in mtDNA are maternally inherited by all the embryos. In theory, one could prevent the inheritance of mitochondrial disorders by means of nuclear transplantation into an enucleated egg from a healthy donor, resulting in one or more embryos which have their *nuclear* DNA from the affected woman and her partner and normal *mtDNA* from the egg donor. There is a lot of confusion, even in the scientific literature, about the question whether this type of nuclear transplantation involves cloning or not. The correct answer depends on the specifics of the strategy to be used.

There are at least three options:

- to transplant the nucleus of the unfertilized egg or oocyte;
- to transplant both pronuclei of the zygote;
- to transplant the nucleus of a blastomere (or the nucleus of several blastomeres).

While the first and second method would not involve the cloning (duplication) of an embryo, the latter approach definitely would. It would, however, not necessarily involve *reproductive* embryo cloning. After all, one could decide to transfer only one embryo thus constructed (even though this strategy would probably decrease the THBR).

Human embryo research (pre-clinical feasibility and safety studies) will be necessary for the development of these different types of REC. Such research is notably controversial. In considering the ethics of human embryo research aiming at the further development of REC, a *preliminary* question is, of course, whether clinical REC as such would be acceptable from a moral point of view. Clearly, if REC cannot be morally justified, pre-clinical research would be unjustified.

Therapeutic cloning

Experts have high expectations of the use of human embryonic stem cells (ESC) - pluripotent cells that give rise to all adult cell types - for transplantation purposes. Currently, research concentrates on ESC obtained from *spare* preimplantation embryos.[9] By culturing these embryos in vitro up to the blastocyst stage (5 days after fertilization), isolating their ESC, and controlling the in vitro differentiation of these cells, scientists hope to be able to produce all sorts of transplants.

From the outset, however, many experts thought that the full therapeutic potential of ESC would depend on TC. This strategy involves the *creation* **of** *embryos* by transplanting nuclei of somatic cells of individual patients into enucleated eggs. ESC isolated from these embryos (clones from the patient) might be grown in vitro to produce 'matched' transplants for patients suffering from all sorts of serious disorders. TC, although not yet practicable, could open the way towards a type of cell (or tissue) replacement therapy that avoids the problems of immune rejection.[10]

According to many experts, TC may well be the most beneficial application of cloning in the human.

What about the ethics?

I will first explore the ethics of REC, more in particular REC in the context of regular IVF, and then comment on the ethics of TC.

Reproductive embryo cloning: ethical aspects

REC can best be evaluated from a moral point of view by making a detour, i.e. by putting REC in the perspective of the paradigm case of human cloning, the reproductive cloning of adults/children. I will, therefore, briefly summarize the ethical debate about (the main objections to) the reproductive cloning of adults/children.. The question, then, becomes: do these objections also apply to REC?

'It is unnatural' The 'argument from nature' is, even though it is often used in debates regarding bioethical issues, questionable. The argument that 'X is wrong because it is unnatural' can only succeed if there is an interpretation of the term '(un)natural' which enables us both to clearly distinguish between natural and unnatural actions/interventions/conditions, *and* to understand why the latter are morally objectionable. It is doubtful whether there are any such interpretations which are convincing. What matters morally are the goals, the means and the consequences of our actions. So, 'the argument from nature' is a non sequitur - from the fact that reproductive cloning by nuclear transfer is unnatural in the human, it does not follow that it is morally unjustified.

'It is an invasion of human dignity' It is not always clear what this objection exactly means: whose dignity is attacked and how?[11] According to Kantian ethics, respect for human dignity requires that a human person is never used *exclusively* as a means. Critics of cloning, however, do not convincingly demonstrate (or even try to demonstrate) that *all* sorts of reproductive cloning would necessarily involve a complete instrumentalization of the future child. Maybe, one can reasonably argue that the objection does apply to some specific cases of cloning. For instance, if one really wants to make a copy (genetic as well as phenotypic) of a highly valued individual (the 'replica' motive), or when one would clone someone in order to use the child for transplantation purposes.

'It is a violation of the right to have a unique genotype' This objection has been convincingly criticized by, amongst others, Brock.[12] A first question, so

he argues, would be whether we do have a right to a unique genotype at all. Critics of cloning probably argue that children have the right to develop a unique *identity*. The view, however, that the clone will not be able to develop its own identity, seems to presume a crude, untenable, genetic determinism - which undermines the validity of the objection. It is important to acknowledge that the parent and its clone will grow up 'in another time, at another place'; the further separated in time, the more different the environment, and the more different the environmental influence on development, character and individuality.

Jonas' version of the objection holds that cloning a human, more in particular the *asynchrony* between the 'original' and the clone, would violate the clone's 'right not to know'[13] a later twin knows, or at least believes to know, too much about himself. It may seem that the clone's life has already been lived by another, that the clone's fate is already determined. The central difficulty in this argument is that the right to ignorance is not violated merely because the later twin is likely to *believe* that his future is already determined, when that belief is clearly false and supported only by the crudest genetic determinism;

> If we know the later twin will falsely believe that his open future has been taken from him as a result of being cloned, even though in reality it has not, then we know that cloning will cause the twin psychological distress, but not that it will violate his right.[14]

Jonas' critique may well be interpreted as a disguised consequentialist objection, pointing to psychosocial harms to the clone.

'Cloning carries substantial medical risks' As animal research shows, (current methods of) cloning results in high numbers of miscarriages and higher perinatal mortality and morbidity rates. Human adult cloning would probably have similar adverse outcomes. Furthermore, clones might be predisposed to decreased life span (due to the progressive shortening of telomeres in older cells). The finding that sheep created through somatic nuclear transfer do have shorter telomeres further increases the latter risk - even though the shorter telomeres have not have had any detectable effects so far.[15]

'Cloning carries substantial psychosocial risks' The asynchrony between the person cloned ('the original') and the later twin could have adverse psychosocial consequences for the latter. After all, the later twin may suffer from perceiving himself, and/or being perceived by others, as some sort of a

'copy' of someone who already exists.

Some commentators consider this type of criticism to be morally irrelevant. They argue that the value of being alive outweighs any disvalue associated with the putative psychosocial harms of cloning. The alternative to coming into existence as a clone of another is not to exist at all. Clearly, so they argue, for the clone existence is to be preferred above non-existence.[16] This rebuttal (the 'argument from non-existence'), however, is controversial. According to the American 'National Advisory Board on Ethics in Reproduction' (NABER), the argument presupposes that children born of cloning are waiting in the void of non-existence to be summoned into existence, and that if they do not receive the call to life, they are harmed. Clearly, there are no non-existent children who could be damaged by not being born.[17] I doubt whether this objection to the argument from non-existence is valid. After all, the argument does not (or at least not necessarily) presume that to refrain from procreation harms any 'children waiting to be conceived'. The argument from non-existence may, however, be flawed for another reason: Those who argue that it is better for a child to have been born, even by cloning, that from his perspective, existence is better than non-existence, make a judgment about a child who already exists - who has *no alternative but death.* The 'psychosocial harm' objection to cloning (or other techniques), however, concerns children who do not yet exist. It is not incoherent to argue that one should refrain from creating children if they would greatly suffer as a result of the procreative method used.

The argument from non-existence would justify almost any harm to befall on future children. I agree with Brock that the psychosocial risks to the clone are more or less speculative, but that the argument from non-existence does not provide a compelling argument to disregard these risks.[18]

For the moment, there is consensus that reproductive adult (or child) cloning would be morally unjustified. The 'medical risk'-objection is, at least for the time being, are overriding. Some objections (e.g. 'it is unnatural') are less convincing or even weak, while others, more in particular the 'psychosocial risk'-argument, need further ethical scrutiny.

What, then, about *the ethics of REC*, more in particular REC in the context of regular IVF?

According to the Additional Protocol of the Convention on Human Rights and Biomedicine,

> Any intervention seeking to create a human being genetically identical to another human being, whether living or dead, is prohibited. (art.1) [19]

This article entails a categorical prohibition of REC. This prohibition is, I think, premature, in view of the fact that there has not been any public debate about the ethics of REC. Furthermore, one may wonder whether art.1, taken literally, does apply to REC at all. After all, REC does not *seek* to create identical twins - its primary aim is to increase the success rate of IVF. Of course, the birth of a monozygotic twin may be the (unintended) consequence of REC - but does that matter morally?

It may be useful to make a comparative analysis of reproductive adult cloning on the one hand and REC on the other hand: Do the objections to adult cloning also apply to REC?

'It is unnatural' This objection is even less convincing if applied to REC. In view of the phenomenon of 'natural' twinning, one might even argue that REC is an *imitation* of nature, at least if one would make only *one* 'copy', and transfer the monozygotic embryos thus obtained in the *same* cycle - a strategy coined 'simple fresh-transfer twinning' by Bonnicksen.[20]

'It is an invasion of human dignity' It is difficult to see how REC aiming at increasing the THBR of IVF could attack human dignity. In any case, REC in the context of regular IVF would not be motivated by the suspect 'replica' motive. In theory, REC could be combined with 'progeny testing', which would involve the storing of cloned embryos while a few are transferred to test their social and personal attributes.[21] The psychosocial and ethical problems inherent in this (hypothetical) scenario do, however, not constitute an objection to the applications of REC just described.

The 'medical risk' objection It is important to discern the two methods of embryo cloning. REC by means of nuclear transfer will probably be less risky than reproductive adult cloning, because (this type of) embryo cloning would involve the transplantation of *'young'* nuclei, which had not yet accumulated DNA-damage, nor have shorter telomeres. It is premature, however, to suggest, as Edwards and Beard do, that cloning from embryonic nuclei is safe.[22] REC by means of blastomere separation may carry less health risks for progeny than nuclear transfer. Clearly, (further) pre-clinical safety studies could contribute to a better understanding of potential risks of both of these methods.

The 'psychosocial harm' objection Psychosocial harms might be easily prevented by avoiding asynchrony between future monozygous twins, (for instance) by a simultaneous transfer of monozygotic 'twin-embryos'. Clearly, a *sequential* transfer resulting in asynchrony between identical twins could involve psychosocial harms. Bonnicksen points especially to the adverse effects of parental expectations or fears:

> If a child is born as a spaced twin pressures on the first born and the second born are possible, as parents wonder why the second one does not turn out like the first one (if the first one is successful) or worry that the second born will turn out like the first born (if the first born is unsuccessful).[23]

Obviously, twins, especially the later twin, could also suffer if their parents would *not* have such expectations or fears. Even if the later twin would not believe in genetic determinism, he may feel that he constantly lives in the shadow of the older twin.

When sequential transfers would result in asynchrony between identical twins, REC would, paradoxically, be similar to reproductive *adult* cloning. The psychosocial risks of asynchrony between identical twins produced by REC could even be greater than the psychosocial risks of cloning adults, as in the first case nature *as well as the environment* ('nurture') would be identical, potentially resulting in greater problems, especially for the second born twin, in developing his own identity.

With regard to REC in the context of regular IVF my tentative conclusions are the following:

- At least some of the moral objections to the reproductive cloning of adults/children do not, or not necessarily, apply to REC;
- There seem to be no valid categorical objections to 'simple fresh-transfer twinning' - the simple case of REC.

The real issue, then, is not whether REC can be morally justified, but *which conditions* should be imposed. According to Bonnicksen, 'simple fresh-transfer twinning' is as far as doctors should go because one should not risk asynchrony between identical twins.[24]   Although I fully agree that a sequential transfer of identical embryos, potentially resulting in asynchrony between monozygotic twins, is ethically more problematic than simple fresh-transfer twinning, I am not yet convinced that risking asynchrony must be avoided. On the one hand it is important to weigh the risk of psychosocial harm to the 'later' twin. On the other hand one should acknowledge that Bonnicksen's proposal (to restrict REC to 'simple fresh-transfer twinning') would substantially decrease the potential clinical value of REC. After all, it would not be possible to reach one of the goals of REC, namely to minimise the burdens of IVF by cryopreserving a set of cloned embryos for transfer in a next cycle.

The potential applications of REC in the context of genetic technologies would raise partly *different* issues (in comparison with REC in the context of regular IVF). *First*, (selective) REC to increase the success rate of IVF/PGD?[25] No doubt, selective REC might be useful in individual cases. It is important, however, to anticipate its potential impact on 'preimplantation selection'. One of the concerns regarding PGD is that PGD will result in a selection of embryos for trivial reasons, especially as it will become possible to test embryos for many characteristics at the same time ('multiplex testing'), and that PGD will eventually allow prospective parents to design the 'perfect' child. According to Schulman and Edwards this last fear is unfounded, as more embryos may be needed to obtain the desired genetic combinations than a women can produce in a lifetime.[26] This rebuttal is convincing - for the moment. It is important, however, to timely acknowledge the potential implications of the *combination* of PGD with new technologies like the in vitro maturation (IVM) of eggs and selective REC. If it becomes possible to create large numbers of embryos by fertilizing large numbers of eggs obtained by IVM (a), and to multiply the embryo which proves to be 'the best' after multiplex testing (b), the 'designer baby' could well become a realistic option in the future. Where to draw the line? What constitutes a sound 'ethics of preimplantation selection'?

Second, nucleus transfer in order to prevent the transmission of mitochondrial disorders. *One* of the methods which could be used (the transplantation of nuclei isolated from blastomeres) would involve embryo cloning. It would, of course, be premature to conclude that, in order to avoid embryo cloning, one of the *other* methods should be investigated. Part of the ethical analysis that is needed is a comparative analysis of the respective pros and cons of the various methods.

Clearly, the ethics of REC in the context of genetic technologies is more complex than the ethics of REC in the context of regular IVF, because the first type of REC is interwoven with other controversial issues, more in particular embryo selection and germ line genetic intervention.

Therapeutic cloning: ethical aspects

The potential benefits of TC are clear: TC might enable the production of 'matched' preimplantation embryos for the treatment of serious disorders. The major ethical problem is that TC involves the production of *embryos* purely for instrumental use. In this respect, TC is similar to the issue of creating embryos for *research* purposes, the neuralgic point in the debate about human embryo research.

While many countries allow the use of spare embryos in research (if some conditions are met), creating embryos for research purposes is much more controversial. The latter is prohibited by the Convention on Human Rights and Biomedicine of the Council of Europe.[27] One may wonder, however, whether there is a fundamental moral difference between on the one hand using spare embryos ('left-overs') in research and on the other hand the generation of embryos for research purposes. Of course, the intention at the moment of fertilization is different - the creation of embryos for research implies their 'instrumentalization' right from the start. Irrespective of their 'origin', however, embryos have the *same* moral status. So, if one accepts the instrumental use of spare embryos (in view of their relatively low moral status), one can hardly object to the creation of embryos for research purposes on the ground that it involves instrumental use. From a consequentialist perspective, an absolute prohibition of creating embryos for research is disputable, because it blocks an adequate pre-clinical risk assessment of some new techniques, like the cryopreservation of eggs, and IVM. In view of the relatively low moral status of the preimplantation embryo it seems reasonable to argue that research on spare embryos as well as creating embryos for research purposes may be morally justified if the research serves important health interests.

The UK's Human Fertilisation and Embryology Act (1990) allows the creation of human embryos for research purposes on some conditions. The Act contains a limitative list concerning the permissible purposes for embryo research. The Act actually states that such research should be limited to 'reproductive matters'. Similarly, the Dutch Minister of Health has announced that future legislation in the Netherlands will allow embryo research only if related to reproductive matters. This policy has been criticized. The Human Fertilisation and Embryology Authority and the Human Genetics Advisory Commission recommended that research directed to TC should be allowed as well.[28] This recommendation is, I think, reasonable. After all, it would be inconsistent to allow embryo research for the development of new *'life giving'* treatments (new types of ART), and at the same time to categorically prohibit the use of preimplantation embryos for research aiming at the development of *'life saving'* technologies.

There is a strong consensus that human embryos may only be used in research if there are *no (good) alternatives*. The same condition should, of course, apply to TC.

According to the literature, there may be various alternatives to TC (and to the use of ESC from spare preimplantation IVF-embryos). It might, for example, be possible to get autologous transplants by directly redifferentiating somatic cells of the patient, thereby circumventing the production of embryos for instrumental use. Furthermore, at least some types of stem cells derived from *adults* seem to have an unexpected versatility. According to recent animal studies, neural stem cells may be able to develop into blood cells.[29] And stem cells from human bone marrow have been reported to generate functional neural cells.[30] If confirmed, adult stem cell versatility could open the way to cell therapies that do not rely on ESC with their ethical entanglements.

It remains to be seen, however, whether adult stem cells can really fulfill the same potential as ESC can. One drawback of adult stem cells is that some seem to lose their ability to divide and differentiate after a time in culture. This short life-span may make them unsuitable for some medical applications. For these and other reasons, many researchers say, adult-derived stem cells are not going to be an exact substitute for ESC.[31] Accordingly, TC might be the best therapeutic option in some cases, for some types of disorders.

While the ethical debate about creating embryos for instrumental use traditionally concentrates on the moral value of the human embryo (reflecting a so-called 'fetalist' perspective), from a *feminist* perspective the issue becomes more complex. Some feminist critics have questioned the acceptability of creating embryos for research out of concern for the autonomy and the interests of the women donating eggs for research.[32] This criticism does, of course, also apply to the creation of embryos for transplantation purposes. After all, in order to obtain eggs, women have to undergo hormone stimulation 'therapy' and invasive medical procedures, which carry some medical risks. Furthermore, so the argument runs, there is a serious risk of exploitation, in view of the temptation to withhold detailed information on risks for fear of losing 'willing' candidate donors of eggs. These feminist concerns are, of course, important, but they can hardly justify an absolute ban on creating pre-implantation embryos for research or transplantation purposes. Firstly, the interests of donors may be sufficiently protected by imposing the condition that medical risks should be minimized, by limiting the numbers of hormone treatments as well as the dosage of hormones given to candidate donors. Of course, a valid informed consent presumes adequate information about potential residual risks. Secondly, the feminist objection seems to be particularly weak with regard to one specific subgroup of candidate-donors: women who may benefit from the new techniques themselves ('auto-donation'). Thirdly, IVM of oocytes might make hormonal treatments (for this purpose) obsolete - it could even imply the access to altogether new 'sources' of research eggs, including aborted female fetuses and cadavers.

Interestingly, some commentators have suggested the use of eggs from *other species* for human TC purposes: nuclei derived from patients' cells could be transplanted into enucleated eggs of, for instance, a cow. Proponents claim that this strategy could circumvent both the feminist as well as the 'fetalist' objections to creating human embryos for instrumental use.[33]   A first question is whether this is a feasible alternative.   As yet, normal development has not been obtained with nuclear transfers between species.   It is, according to a recent review article, unlikely that animal eggs could be used as an alternative to human eggs as recipients for human nuclei.[34]   The second question is, of course, whether the claim, that this alternative (if feasible) would avoid the ethical problems inherent in the creation of human embryos for TC, is valid.   Obviously, the feminist critique would not apply to the use of animals as egg donors.   But does this alternative also avoid the 'fetalist' objection?   An affirmative answer presumes that one can convincingly argue that the 'interspecies' embryo constructed by means of this combination is not a *human* embryo.[35]   In view of the fact that all of the nuclear DNA of these embryos will be inherited from their human 'parents', I doubt whether this argument is valid.

Conclusion

REC, more in particular 'simple fresh-transfer twinning', can be accepted from a moral point of view.   The categorical prohibition of REC entailed in the Council of Europe's Additional Protocol is, therefore, unjustified. In view of both the potential clinical value of REC and the relatively low moral status of the preimplantation embryo, pre-clinical research aiming at evaluating the feasibility and risks of REC can be morally acceptable.

At the same time, REC raises issues which need further debate. Relevant for regular IVF is especially whether sequential transfers of identical embryos, potentially resulting in asynchrony between identical twins (or triplets), could be morally justified.   Furthermore, the potential application of REC in the context of genetic technologies is interwoven with complex moral issues regarding embryo selection and germ line genetic intervention.

In view of the relatively low moral, the principle of proportionality implies that if we accept the creation of embryos for research aiming at the further development of ART, we should definitely allow the creation of embryos for the production of life saving transplants - at least if there are no good alternatives.

For the moment, there seems to be a strong consensus regarding this latter condition. This consensus, however, may well prove to be superficial and/or tottering. Recent publications mention various potential (future) alternatives for TC (and for the use of ESC obtained from spare IVF-embryos). In view of these potential alternatives, we need to address some thorny questions.

a) Do we really think than *any* alternative is better, from a moral point of view, than using human embryos? Is, for instance, xenotransplantation morally less problematic - even though this alternative carries unknown risks for public health? And is the use of adult stem cells definitely to be preferred, even if invasive and risky procedures may be necessary to obtain these cells?

b) Do we really think that *all* potential alternatives should be studied in depth before the use of human embryos may be considered, even those alternatives which are highly theoretical (according to most of the experts)?

c) Last, but not least: what if most of the experts think that the development of specific alternatives will probably take substantially more time than the development of TC? Are we, then, obliged, to delay studies involving human embryos/ESC - and to take the risk that life saving treatment may come too late for some patients?

Clearly, different views about how to proceed, and about the precise implications of the principle that human embryos can be used instrumentally only as a last resort, not only reflect different scientific opinions and expectations, but also different value judgements, more in particular different views on the moral status of the preimplantation embryo. If we think that the status of the human preimplantation embryo is (rather) low, and that the development of new life saving treatments is of utmost importance, we may well conclude that research on human ESC and TC should not be restricted, and that stem cell specialists should be able to study both adult and embryonic stem cells - even though in the long run 'embryo saving' alternatives may prove to be perfect substitutes.

In any case, if the alternatives prove to be of limited value, the prospect of TC may well function as a catalyst for allowing the creation of embryos for instrumental use in various European nations.

Notes

1   Wilmut I, Schnieke AE, McWhir J, Kind AJ, Campbell KHS. 'Viable offspring derived from fetal and adult mammalian cells'. *Nature* (1997), vol. 385, pp. 810-813.

2   Wert G de. (1998) 'Kloneren bij de mens: ethische reflecties bij mogelijke toepassingen'. Verslag Symposium Kloneren. KNAW/NIBI, pp. 33-36.

3   According to the UK Human Genetics Advisory Commission and the Human Fertilisation and Embryology Authority, the term 'cloning' carries an automatic stigma for many because of its association with imagery such as that portrayed in Brave New World. To avoid this confusion, these committees replaced 'therapeutic cloning' by 'therapeutic use of cell nucleus transfer' Cf.: Human Genetics Advisory Commission, Human Fertilisation and Embryology Authority. Cloning issues in reproduction, science and medicine. 1998.

4   Jones HW, Edwards RG, Seidel GE. (1994) 'On attempts at cloning in the human.' *Fertility and Sterility*; vol 64, pp. 423-426.

5   Gosden R. (1999) 'Designing babies'. *The brave new world of reproductive technology.* Freeman.

6   Cohen J. Tomkin G. (1994) 'The science, fiction and reality of embryo cloning'. *Kennedy Institute of Ethics Journal*; vol. 4, pp. 193-203.

7   Wolf DP. (1997) 'Genetic manipulation by nuclear transfer'. Special Issue: Abstracts from Second International Symposium on Preimplantation Genetics. *Journal of Assisted Reproduction Genetics,* vol. 14, p. 480.

8   Pembrey M. (1992) 'Embryo therapy: is there a clinical need?' In: Bromham D, Dalton M, Jackson J, et al., eds., *Ethics in reproductive medicine.* London: Springer Verlag, pp. 11-20.

9   Thomson JA, Itskovitz-Eldor J, Shapiro SS, et al. (1998) 'Embryonic stem cells lines derived from human blastocysts'. *Science,* vol. 282, pp. 1145-1147.

10   Gurdon JB, Colman A. (1999) 'The future of cloning'. *Nature,* vol. 402, pp.743-746.

11   Harris J. (1997) '"Goodbye Dolly?" The ethics of human cloning'. *Journal of Medical Ethics,* vol.23, pp. 353-360.

12   Brock DW. (1998) 'Cloning human beings: An assessment of the ethical issues pro and con'. In: Nussbaum MC, Sunstein CR, eds., *Clones and clones. Facts and fantasies about human cloning.* Norton & Company, New York, London, pp. 141-164.

13   Jonas H. (1982) 'Lasst uns einen Menschen klonieren. Betrachtungen zur Aussicht genetischer Versuche mit uns selbst'. *Scheidewege,* vol. 12, pp. 462-449.

14   Brock, *op. cit.*

15   Shiels PG, Kind AJ, Campbell KHS, et al. (1999) 'Analysis of telomere lengths in cloned sheep'. *Nature,* vol. 399, pp. 316-317; Gurdon and Colman, o.c.

16   Chadwick R. (1982) 'Cloning'. *Philosophy,* vol. 57, pp. 201-209; Burley J, Harris J. Human (1999) 'Cloning and child welfare.' *Journal of Medical Ethics,* vol. 25, pp.108-113.

17   National Advisory Board on Ethics in Reproduction. (1994) 'Report on human cloning through embryo splitting: an amber light.' *Kennedy Institute of Ethics Journal,* vol. 4, pp. 251-282.

18   Brock, *op. cit.*

19   Council of Europe (1997)Additional protocol to the Convention for the protection of human rights and dignity of the human being with regard to the application of biology and medicine on the prohibition of cloning human beings.

20 Bonnicksen AL. (1995) 'Ethical and policy issues in human embryo twinning'. *Cambridge Quarterly of Healthcare Ethics*, vol 4, pp. 268-284.

21 Edwards RG, Beard HK. (1998) 'How identical would cloned children be? An understanding essential to the ethical debate'. *Human Reproduction* Update, vol. 4, pp. 791-811.

22 Edwards, Beard, *op. cit.*

23 Bonnicksen, *op. cit.*

24 *Id.*

25 For an ethical analysis of PGD see: Wert G de. (1999) 'Ethics of assisted reproduction: the case of preimplantation genetic diagnosis'. In: Fauser BCJM, Rutherford AJ, Strauss JF III, Steirteghem A van, eds., *Molecular Biology in Reproductive Medicine.*: Parthenon Publishers, New York/London, pp. 433-448.

26 Schulman JD, Edwards RG. (1996) 'Preimplantation diagnosis is disease control, not eugenics'. *Human Reproduction,* vol. 11, pp. 463-664.

27 Council of Europe. Convention on Human Rights and Biomedicine. Strasbourg, 1996.

28 Human Genetics Advisory Commission, Human Fertilisation and Embryology Authority, *op. cit.*

29 Bjornson CRR, Rietze RL, Reynolds BA, et al. (1999) 'Turning brain into blood: a hematopoietic fate adopted by adult neural stem cells in vivo'. *Science,* vol., pp. 283:534-537.

30 Azizi SA, et al. (1998) 'Engraftment and migration of human bone marrow stromal cells implanted in the brains of albino rats'. *Proceedings of the National Academy of Sciences. USA,* vol. 95, pp. 3908-3913.

31 Vogel G. (2000) 'Can old cells learn new tricks?' *Science*, vol. 287, pp. 1418-1419.

32 Gerrand N. (1993) 'Creating embryos for research'. *Journal of Applied Philosophy*, vol 10, pp. 175-187.

33 Lanza RP, Cibelli JB, West MD. (1999) 'Human therapeutic cloning' *Nature Medicine,* vol. 5, pp. 975-977.

34 Gurdon, Colman, *op. cit.*

35 Massachusetts researchers reported that they had already transferred nuclei from human somatic cells into enucleated bovine oocytes to form preimplantation embryos. According to Annas et al., the protocol (if one existed) was not reviewed by the University of Massachusetts' local Institutional Review Board. It is according to these authors, a crime in Massachusetts to use any living fetus, which the statute defines as including an embryo, for research. Annas et al. explain the failure to submit the research protocol to a Review Board by the fact that the researchers were veterinarians and not physicians. (Annas GJ, Caplan A, Elias S. (1999) 'Stem cell politics, ethics and medical progress'. *Nature Medicine* vol. 5, pp. 1339-1341.) An alternative explanation is that the researchers did not consider these 'units' to be **human** embryos.

Part III
LAW

10 Overview: Legislative Approaches

JENNIFER GUNNING

Background

It is now well over 20 years since the treatment of infertility by means of in vitro fertilization became a reality. But it is 30 years since the first human egg was fertilized in vitro, an event that momentarily stirred up a frisson of concern around the world. Speaking to the science and technology panel of the US House of Representatives Committee on Science and Astronautics in 1971 James Watson, Nobel Prize winner and co-discoverer of the structure of DNA, said:

> We must assume that techniques for the in vitro manipulation of human eggs are likely to be general medical practice, capable of routine performance in many major countries in some 10 to 20 years.

and

> This matter is far too important to be left solely in the hands of the scientific and medical communities. The belief that surrogate mothers and clonal babies are inevitable because science moves forward ... represents a form of laissez faire nonsense dismally reminiscent of the creed that American business if left to itself will solve everybody's problems. Just as the success of a corporate body in making money need not set the human condition ahead, neither does every scientific advance automatically make our lives more meaningful.

Of course, Watson was right. Within 20 years of his comment assisted conception, based on in vitro fertilization, was widely available across the world and not only in the major nations. Despite his warning, the laissez faire attitude to the regulation of these new reproductive technologies has continued to prevail, particularly in the USA.

The birth of the first IVF child in 1978 provided the stimulus for activity in a number of countries to consider the ethics of human embryo research and the clinical use of IVF. But, over the years, much discussion has resulted in little legislation and even less regulation of clinical practice. For instance, currently only 7 of the 15 EU Member States have legislation addressing IVF and, of these, only 3 have regulatory bodies overseeing clinical provision.

National legislation

The route to legislation has varied from country to country but the principal focus has been the status of the human embryo and the ethics of human embryo research. Some countries have national ethics committees, standing bodies who are charged with giving opinions on biomedical issues. The Danish National Council of Ethics, for instance, was established specifically to advise the Danish government on assisted reproduction and genetic engineering and had a major influence on the subsequent Danish legislation. Its remit has since extended to other issues in medical ethics such as death criteria and xenotransplantation. Governments in other countries have chosen to establish specific committees of enquiry to make recommendations on human embryo research and IVF. Examples are the Benda Committee in Germany and the Warnock Committee in the United Kingdom. These committees also informed subsequent legislation though the delays to implementation were different. The German government acted relatively swiftly to enact restrictive legislation following the Benda report. Five years elapsed between the Warnock Report and the Human Fertilisation and Embryology Act in the UK.

The legislation so far enacted in Europe falls into three categories. Into the first category fall those countries that have laws forbidding all research on human embryos. These include Germany (Embryo Protection Act, 13 December 1990), Austria (Act No. 275, Reproductive Medicine Law, 1992), France (Law No. 94-654 of 29 July 1994), Norway (Law No. 68 on Artificial Fertilization, 12 June 1987) and Switzerland specifically or by implication through a number of individual cantonal laws. The Austrian law does allow examination and treatment of embryos if such action is necessary to achieve a pregnancy and an amendment to the French law (Decree No. 97-613, 27 May 1997 on Studies Conducted on Human Embryos in vitro) provides that studies on human embryos in vitro may be carried out only to offer direct advantage to the embryo concerned.

The second category covers those countries which, while specifically prohibiting the creation of embryos for research, allow research on embryos which are surplus to a therapeutic program. These include Estonia (Law of 11 July 1997 on Artificial Embryos), Hungary (Act No. CLIV 1997 Chapter VII on Extraordinary Human Reproduction Treatment, on Research on Embryos and Gametes and on Sterilization) and Spain (Law No. 35 of 22 November 1988 on Assisted Reproduction Procedures). The Hungarian law specifically prohibits the reimplantation of embryos which have been the subject of experiment. The implementation of the Spanish law was delayed until 1997 because it was subject to a challenge through the Constitutional Court.

Three countries enacted legislation which did not specifically prohibit the creation of embryos for research and specifically allowed human embryo research. These are the United Kingdom (Human Fertilisation and Embryology Act 1990), Sweden (Law No. 115 of 14 March 1991 concerning Measures for the Purposes of Research or Treatment in connection with Fertilized Human Oocytes) and Denmark (Law No. 460 of 10 June 1997 on Artificial Fertilization in connection with Medical Treatment, Diagnosis and Research). The laws in the UK, Sweden and Denmark all prohibit the return to the uterus of embryos which have been the subject of research.

Since passing its 1997 Act, Denmark has signed and ratified the European Convention on Human Rights and Biomedicine without a reservation on Article 18 on human embryo research. This means that future embryo research in Denmark will be restricted to surplus embryos. Sweden has signed but not ratified the Convention and the UK has neither signed nor ratified it. This could leave the UK as the only country in Europe having legislation allowing the creation of embryos for research. Though there are countries, such as Belgium, which have neither signed the Convention nor enacted legislation.

But the enactment of legislation does not necessarily mean that the provision of assisted reproduction services is regulated to ensure best practice. In fact, some laws may encourage the reverse. The German law does not allow the transfer of more than three embryos in one treatment cycle nor does it allow the fertilization of more eggs than may be transferred in a treatment cycle. This puts constraints on doctors when the factors contributing to embryo quality are still poorly understood and has a negative impact on the chances of success for patients. Moreover, the necessity for patients to undergo several cycles of hormonal stimulation, with its accompanying risks, is likely to be increased. Elsewhere the trend is to collect a larger number of eggs in one cycle and freezing the surplus for future treatments. The law in Norway prohibits the freezing and storage of unfertilized oocytes but the problems with egg freezing may soon be overcome by research. Stored eggs are less likely to present an ethical problem than stored embryos yet embryos are allowed to be stored for one year in Norway.

Legislation is often unable to take account of unforeseen or unintended consequences. If, rather than setting up a framework, laws are too prescriptive they may set up a barrier to progress or require frequent amendment. The fact that the German Embryo Protection Act requires all fertilized eggs to be returned to the womb means that preimplantation genetic diagnosis (PGD) is not possible in Germany. The whole purpose of PGD is to detect embryos affected by a serious genetic disorder so that they need not be returned to the womb thus avoiding the need to terminate an affected pregnancy or the birth of a child with a serious disease. German couples seeking this procedure must find it outside Germany.

In only three countries is there statutory regulation of the provision of assisted conception services. In the United Kingdom the 1990 Act established a regulatory body, the Human Fertilisation and Embryology Authority. Its remit and method of operation are described by Martin Johnson in chapter 12. Although the Netherlands have yet to legislate on human embryo research, a law has been in force since 1988 regulating ART facilities (Decree of 11 August 1988 amending subsection1 of Section 1 and subsection 1 of Section 18 of the law of 1971 on hospital facilities). This requires laboratories and centers involved in IVF and IVF treatment procedures to be licensed by the Minister of Welfare, Public Health and Culture. In France an arrêté of 12 January 1999 requires clinics and laboratories involved in medically assisted reproduction to adhere to a detailed code of good practice.

Of course, the lack of statutory regulation does not necessarily mean that there is no regulation. In most countries where assisted conception services are available there is some form of professional self-regulation. The advantages of professional self-regulation over statutory legislation are mainly its broader acceptance among those to whom it is addressed and its greater flexibility. However, it can be criticized for lacking democratic legitimacy and control. Professional self-regulation runs the risk of an overemphasis on medical or biological aspects while sociological aspects may be neglected. Those involved in this regulatory process are generally fellow medical professionals and they may be too close to professional practice to take an entirely objective view. However, in some countries such as Greece, where IVF treatment has flourished since 1985, there is no form of regulation.

European Convention on Human Rights and Biomedicine

After many years of gestation the European Convention on Human Rights and Biomedicine opened for signature in Oviedo, Spain, on 4 April 1997. It was immediately signed by 23 of the 40 Member States of the Council of Europe. By September 1999 the Convention had been signed by 28 Member States and ratified by six (see Table 1 at the end of this chapter), allowing it to come into to force on 1 December 1999. Of those countries which have ratified the Convention, Denmark, Greece, San Marino, Slovakia, Slovenia and Spain, only two, Denmark and Spain have legislation on assisted conception.

Following the publicity surrounding the cloning of Dolly the sheep, in 1998 the Council of Europe published an Additional Protocol to the Convention on the Prohibition of Cloning Human Beings. It was opened for signature in Paris on 12 January 1998. It was open for signature only to those countries which had already signed the Convention. The Protocol was immediately signed by 19 countries. Articles 1 and 2 of the Protocol are to be regarded as additional articles of the Convention and are as follows:

1. Any intervention seeking to create a human being genetically identical to another human being, whether living or dead, is prohibited.
2. For the purpose of this article, the term human being "genetically identical" to another human being means a human being sharing with another the same nuclear gene set.

Article 18 of the Convention requires the adequate protection of the embryo in cases where the signatory country allows research on embryos in vitro but the article prohibits the creation of embryos for research. Countries already having a law in force, which permits the creation of embryos for research, before signing the Convention, are allowed a reservation on article 18 on ratification (article 36). The majority of those countries which have signed the Convention either have no relevant legislation or do not allow the creation of embryos for research. Some countries, such as the Netherlands and Finland are still debating the ethics of the creation of embryos for research and may find themselves in a quandary when it comes to legislation.

Although article 18 of the Convention requires adequate protection of the embryo, this is not defined. It is reported that this has been left deliberately unclear to allow flexibility of interpretation. However, an interpretation could be sought from the European Court of Human Rights.

Currently a protocol on article 18 is in preparation. This should provide some elaboration of the general principles underpinning the article.

Table 10.1 Signatories to the European Convention on Human Rights and biomedicine

Country	Date of signature	Date of ratification
Croatia	07.05.1999	
Cyprus	30.09.1998	
Czech Republic	24.06.1998	
Denmark	04.04.1997	10.08.1999
Estonia	04.04.1997	
Finland	04.04.1997	
France	04.04.1997	
Greece	04.04.1997	06.10.1998
Hungary	07.05.1999	
Iceland	04.04.1997	
Italy	04.04.1997	
Latvia	04.04.1997	
Lithuania	04.04.1997	
Luxembourg	04.04.1997	
Moldova	04.04.1997	
The Netherlands	04.04.1997	
Norway	04.04.1997	
Poland	07.05.1999	
Portugal	04.04.1997	
Romania	04.04.1997	
San Marino	04.04.1997	20.03.1998
Slovakia	04.04.1997	15.01.1998
Slovenia	04.04.1997	05.11.1998
Spain	04.04.1997	01.09.1999
Sweden	04.04.1997	
Switzerland	07.05.1999	
Former Yugoslav Republic of Macedonia	04.04.1997	
Turkey	04.04.1997	

11 Legal Approaches: France

PASCAL KAMINA

Assisted conception in France was regulated in detail for the first time by Act No. 94-654 of July 29 1994 relating to the gift and use of elements and products of the human body, to medically assisted procreation and to prenatal diagnosis, which, with two other Acts of 1994 (Act n°94-548 of July 1, 1994 relating to the processing of personal data for purpose of health research, Act n°94-653 of July 29, 1994 relating to the respect of the human body), form the so-called French *"bioethics laws"*. [1]

This Act of July 29 1994:

- determines the conditions applicable to the gift of gametes and to associated activities;
- sets the conditions for access to assisted conception technologies and regulates these activities;
- provides for criminal administrative sanctions to these rules; and
- deals with some consequences of the use of assisted conception techniques, such as filiation or the fate of extra embryos.

It does not, however, address expressly the status of the embryo.

Article 21 provides for its re-examination by Parliament within 5 years after its entry into force, after an assessment by the Parliamentary Office for Assessment of Scientific and Technological Choices. The assessment was made difficult in some fields by delays in the adoption of some of the 32 implementing decrees contemplated in the Act: in particular, the decree fixing the conditions for authorisation of embryo studies was issued only in May 27, 1997; the decree fixing the conditions for authorisation of institutions undertaking preimplantion diagnosis, in March 24, 1998.

In February 1999 the Parliamentary Office for Assessment of Scientific and Technological Choices adopted its report. As a last step before the reform, the French Conseil d'Etat (supreme administrative court and state legal advisory body) remitted to the Prime Minister a report in November 1999 entitled *The Bioethics Laws: 5 years after*) including several proposals for a new text.

At the time of this article, a bill is in preparation and should be presented to the Parliament.

Overview of the regime of assisted conception and embryo research in France

The main features of French law, deriving from the Act of 1994, are as follows:

A wide definition of "Assisted Conception"

Under article L 152-1 of the French Code of Public Health (Code de la santé publique) (CPH), as modified by a law of July 29, 1994, Medical Assistance to Procreation *(Assistance Médicale à la Procréation) is defined as:

> clinical and biological practices allowing conception in vitro, the transfer of embryos and artificial insemination, all techniques with equivalent effect allowing procreation outside the natural process...

The definition was drafted widely enough to encompass new techniques such as ICSI.

Beneficiaries of assisted conception techniques

Article L. 152-2 of the CPH provides that:

> The man and the woman forming the couple must be alive, of an age to procreate, married or able to provide evidence of a communal life of at least 2 years and consenting prior to the insemination or transfer of the embryo.

In doing so, the article enshrines the common practice of the CECOS (Center for Study and Conservation of Eggs and Sperm) before its adoption. Assisted conception is established in order to answer to the parental wish of a *couple formed by a man and a woman.* As a consequence, it is illegal and a criminal offence to provide AMP to an homosexual couple or to a single person. If the couple does not have to be married, the risks of fraud were discussed in parliament and resulted in a specific requirement of a communal of life of at least 2 years for unmarried couples.

The requirement that the couple must be of procreative age is not further specified. The appreciation is left to the medical doctor.

The two conditions that the couple must be *alive* and *consenting* are linked: the consent (which must be immediate), is of living persons.

Therefore, post mortem inseminations and embryo transfers are equally prohibited. This assimilation was criticised during parliamentary debates.

In the event of death, the surviving spouse or member is consulted in writing on the point to know if they consent that the stored embryos be transferred to another couple (CPH, art. L. 152-4 al 2). But the law does not specify the fate of the embryos if the transfer is refused.

Receiving couples must conform to the same conditions as beneficiary couples.

Indications for assisted conception

The Act provides for only two AMP indications, which confirm the previous practice:

- Infertility of the couple, which must have a pathological (i.e. not natural - e.g. age) origin and must have been medically diagnosed (CPH, art. L. 152-2).
- Risk of transmission of a disease "of a particular gravity" to the child (CPH, art. L. 152-2). This possibility validates *ipso facto* the selection of gametes for this purpose. The disease does not have to be impossible to cure.

The Code also provides for the circumstances in which in vitro conception can be used. Article L. 152-3 of the CPH states that an embryo can be obtained only in the context and according to the aims of assisted conception as defined in article L. 152-2. In order to reinforce these provisions, the Code prohibits in vitro conception of human embryos for study, research or experimental purposes (art. L.152-8), and the conception of human embryos for commercial or industrial purposes (art. L.152-7, but this last prohibition is not limited to in vitro conception).

Article L.152-3 further adds that an embryo cannot be conceived with gametes which do not originate from at least one of the members of the couple. In other terms, the law prohibits the double gift of sperm and oocytes (both members of the couple unfertile). For these couples, AMP has to be performed through the reception of donor embryos.

Regime of assisted conception

In all authorised premises or laboratories, the AMP must be performed under the responsibility of a practitioner authorised to this effect (CPH, art.

L.159-9). Artificial insemination can be performed in a medical office.

The law provides for several compulsory preliminary conversations with members of a multidisciplinary team, which will assess the motivation of the couple and check that it meets the conditions for AMP. In practice, the consultation of a psychologist or a psychiatrist is commonplace (this consultation is compulsory in case of recourse to a third party donor). The aim of these conversations is also to inform the couple on the possibilities of success and failure, and of the painful aspect of assisted conception techniques. The couple is given documentation describing the techniques and including information on the legislative and regulatory provisions relating to AMP, but also to adoption. A period of reflection of one month follows the last conversation, which can be extended by the practitioner. If the couple still wants to proceed with AMP, it must confirm its request in writing.

The Code sets specific rules for in vitro conception and for the storage and transfer of embryos. The two members of the couple can decide in writing the fertilization of a number of oocytes which can result in the storage of embryos for the realisation of their parental wish. There is no limitation on the number of oocytes to be fertilized in vitro, and no limitation on the number of embryos to be transferred.

Conservation of embryos

The possibility granted to the couple to decide on the fertilization in vitro of several oocytes can lead to extra embryos. These embryos can be stored in order to realise later the parental wish of the couple "within a 5 year period" (CPH, art. L.152-3). This duration is not a limit for the conservation of embryos. During this period, the couple can give up their project. They are consulted each year on this matter. But the abandonment by the couple does not involve an end to the storage or the conservation of embryos (or their destruction). The couple who want to withdraw their parental wish within 5 years can only consent to the transfer of the embryos to another couple.

However, by way of exception, the embryos conceived before entry into force of the law can be destroyed at the end of the five years period, if they are not the subject of a parental wish or if their reception by another couple is impossible.

Use of the embryo by another couple

The donation of an embryo is subject to a judicial decision, and to the prior written consent of the originating couple. The judge must control that the receiving couple meets the conditions for AMP. He can also investigate the future familial, educational and psychological environment of the child to be. The intent of Parliament was to create a procedure close to adoption.

The donation is subject to strict anonymity. However, for therapeutic need, a medical doctor can have access to non-identifying information concerning the couple that gave up the embryo.

The donation cannot be remunerated.

Donation of gametes

The regime is the same for sperm and oocytes. The donor must be a member of a couple which already has offspring (CPH, art. L. 673-2). Consent must be obtained in writing from the man and woman in both couples. The donating couple cannot waive its consent, once gametes have been obtained. The donation must be free. There are strict rules of sanitary safety. The law also provides for complete anonymity (except for therapeutic needs, as described).

The realisation of assisted conception with donated gametes has a subsidiary nature: Article L. 152-6 provides that it must be performed as an "ultimate indication", when assisted conception within the couple cannot succeed. The consent of the treated couple is more formal as it takes the form of a declaration in court.

Administrative and health services framework

The decree of May 6, 1995 relating to AMP activities distinguishes between:

- *Clinical activities*, which can only be performed by private or public hospitals, except artificial insemination, which can be performed in a medical doctor's office.
- *Biological activities*, which can usually only be performed in public hospitals and laboratories (laboratoires d'analyses de biologie médicale).

Be they clinical or biological, AMP activities are subject to authorisation (with the exception of artificial insemination). The activities are placed under the responsibility of an agreed practitioner. The authorisation is granted by the Ministry of Public Health after opinion by a specialised national commission (Commission nationale de médecine et de biologie de la reproduction et du diagnostic prénatal). This authorisation is subject to conditions of qualification and is granted for 5 years.

The Act prohibits the remuneration of the medical act of obtaining, processing, conservation and transfer of gametes (CPH, art. L. 673-5).

Embryo research and preimplantation diagnosis

Article L. 152-8 of the CPH provides:

> The conception in vitro of human embryos for study, research or experimental purpose is prohibited.
>
> All experimentation on the embryo is prohibited.
>
> Exceptionally, the man and the woman forming the couple can accept that research be performed on their embryos.
>
> Their decision is expressed in writing.
>
> These studies must have a medical finality and cannot harm the embryo.
>
> They can only be performed after agreement by the commission mentioned in article L.184-3 hereunder [National Commission on Medicine, Reproductive Biology and Prenatal Diagnosis] under the conditions defined by decree.
>
> The commission makes public each year the list of the institutions where these studies are performed, and their objectives.

As a general rule, all experimentation on the embryo is prohibited. However, research can be authorised exceptionally by the couple, providing it has a medical purpose and it cannot harm the embryo. The scope of this provision is specified by a decree of May 27, 1997. Concerning the *medical purpose or finality*, the decree specifies that the research must

(i)   present a direct advantage of the embryo concerned (in particular with a view to increasing its chances of successful implantation), or

(ii)   contribute to the improvement of AMP techniques, in reproduction physiology and pathology.

However, the decree specifies that research *harms* the embryo when it has the effect, or when there is a risk, that it modifies its genetic structure or alters its developing capacities. This language excludes in practice all invasive acts on the embryo.

Preimplantion diagnosis is authorised only exceptionally and under strict conditions fixed by article L. 162-17 of the CPH:

- certification, by a medical doctor practising in a multidisciplinary prenatal diagnosis center, that the couple may give birth to a child with a genetic disease of a particular gravity and known as not curable at the moment of the diagnosis.
- prior identification, with one of the parents, of the anomalies responsible for such a disease
- written consent of the parents
- purpose of the diagnosis, which must be only the identification of the disease and the means to prevent and treat it.

The implementing decree was only issued in March 1998.

Cloning

The Bioethics Acts do not expressly prohibit reproductive cloning. However, the Conseil d'Etat and the National Consultative Ethics Committee consider that article 16-4 of the Civil code includes already a *de jure* prohibition of reproductive cloning:

No one can attempt to alter the integrity of the human species.

All eugenic practices leading to the organisation of the selection of persons is prohibited.

Without prejudice to the research leading to the prevention and treatment of genetic diseases, no change can be made to genetic characteristics with a view to the modification of the descendants of a person.

Also, the provisions of the CPH relating to AMP seem incompatible with cloning techniques which cannot be considered "procreative" methods and which could not comply with the rules on embryo experimentation and research.

The assessment of the law and the proposals for reform

As mentioned, the Act of July 29, 1994 provides for its re-examination by

Parliament within 5 years after its entry into force. At the time of this article, a bill was still not presented to Parliament.

The French Conseil d'Etat remitted in November 1999 to the Prime Minister its report entitled *The bioethics laws: five years after*. The main proposals for reform are as follows:

Reproductive cloning

The Conseil d'Etat first affirms that the re-examination of the Act of July 29, 1994, should be the occasion to affirm the express prohibition of reproductive cloning for humans (within article 16-4 of the Civil code, quoted above).

Embryo research

The Conseil d'Etat proposes to authorise, under a strict monitoring, research on *in vitro* embryos. The principles would be as follows:

- Only frozen *in vitro* embryos which are not the object of a parental project and which cannot be received by another couple, and embryos that are considered non viable, could be the subject of research.
- Embryos subject to research could not be implanted.
- Embryo research would be subject to prior authorisation by an ad hoc authority.

The Conseil d'Etat leaves open the question of knowing whether research should be limited to research on the cells of an embryo or should encompass, as well, research with a view to improving the efficiency of AMP techniques.

Definition of AMP

The Conseil d'Etat proposes to exclude ovarian stimulation techniques from the provisions of articles L. 152-2 and L. 152-9 of the CPH and to submit them to a regime close to the one of artificial insemination.

Finalities of AMP

The Conseil d'Etat proposes

- to modify article L. 152-2 of the CPH to provide that it is possible to obtain and store gametes before a sterilising treatment, with the consent of the concerned person; and
- to provide that AMP is open to couples in which there exists a risk of transmission of a disease of a particular gravity from one member to another (in order to cover the risk of transmission of HIV).

In vitro conception of embryos

The Conseil d'Etat proposes to prohibit a couple from performing a new cycle of in vitro conception if they have frozen embryos in good condition allowing an implantation.

Fate of embryos without parental project

The Conseil d'Etat proposes the following scheme:

A couple which has decided to produce and store extra embryos is consulted each year on their fate:

- if the couple cannot be found or does not answer, the embryos are destroyed after a 5 year period;
- if the couple answers, and the woman is not of procreative age, the couple can only choose to donate the embryo to allocate it to research or to have it destroyed;
- if the woman is of procreative age, and the couple has a parental project, the embryos are stored, even after 5 years;
- if the couple no longer has a parental project, the couple can only chose to donate the embryo, to allocate it to research or to have it destroyed.

Post mortem transfers of embryos

The Conseil d'Etat proposes to authorise the transfer of embryos post mortem under the condition of a formal consent expressed by both members of the couple before the death of the spouse. The woman will be able to request the transfer of the embryos at the minimum three months and at the maximum one year after the death of the husband or partner. The attempt to implant the embryo would have to be performed before the expiry of an 18 months period after the death. Filiation and succession rules will have to be adapted.

Donation of gametes

The Conseil d'Etat proposes to extend the conditions associated with the donor by providing that the donor must be a parent but is not necessarily member of a couple at the time of the donation. If he lives in a couple without the child but with a new spouse or partner, it would be possible either to exclude the possibility of a donation, or to ask for the consent of the other partner. A donation should be revoked at any time before the use of the gametes.

New AMP techniques

The Conseil d'Etat proposes to submit the clinical application of any new AMP technique to a prior authorisation of the Authority which is in charge of the control of assisted procreation.

Note

1   See also Act n°88-1138 of December 1988 relating to the protection of persons subject of biomedical research.

12 The Regulation of Human Embryo Research in the UK: What Implications for Therapeutic Research?

MARTIN H. JOHNSON

Introduction

In the United Kingdom, research on human embryos and on human gametes used in studies on the process of fertilization is lawful but regulated. The Human Fertilisation and Embryology Act (HFE Act) of 1990 (HFEA, 1990) set up a regulatory body, the Human Fertilisation and Embryology Authority (HFEA), which since 1991 has had a statutory responsibility for administering the Act.

The HFE Act's central concern is with the creation, manipulation, keeping, storage (including cryostorage) and use of human embryos in vitro. An embryo is defined as an egg in the process of fertilization, and so the HFE Act effectively covers the mixing of gametes. It therefore regulates, in addition to research on human embryos, the clinical use of those Assisted Reproductive Technologies (ARTs) which involve the actual or intended creation of an in vitro human embryo from human gametes. These include in vitro fertilization and embryo transfer (IVF-ET), intra-cytoplasmic sperm injection (ICSI), and preimplantation genetic diagnosis (PGD). Not included are gamete intra-fallopian transfer (GIFT: unless donor gametes are used, see below), recovery or storage of immature gametes unless or until they are matured in vitro, or surrogacy (unless either embryo transfer or gamete donation clinically is involved - and see below).

In addition to its regulation of the therapeutic and research use of human embryos in vitro, the HFE Act was also used to update and codify the legal regulation of gamete donation clinically, whether or not in the process embryos are created in vitro. It is under this section of the HFE Act that GIFT using donor gametes is regulated. If gametes are taken with the intent of their possible use in clinical donation, then their recovery, manipulation, storage (including cryostorage) and use come within the HFE Act. Regulation applies whether or not the intended use of the gametes is by the donor themselves or some other party. Immature germ cells which are not yet gametes are not covered by the HFE Act. Thus, testicular biopsies from immature males and ovarian biopsies that do not include oocytes in meiotic division are not covered, but spermatids whether round or elongated are. The 1990 Act also amended the Surrogacy Arrangements Act of 1985 to make surrogacy arrangements unenforceable and to change the meaning of "surrogate mother" from that applying under the 1985 Act.

The HFE Act was passed after an extended period of public and political debate and consultation that followed the Warnock Report. During this interim period a professional self-regulatory body, the Voluntary (later renamed Interim) Licensing Authority (VLA) was set up jointly by the Medical Research Council (MRC) and the Royal College of Obstetricians and Gynaecologists (RCOG). This body had lay members and a lay chair, in addition to representatives from the relevant scientific and medical communities. Much of the detailed legislation in the HFE Act was influenced by the experience of this interim regulatory body. (For more details on the working of the VLA, on the background to the legislation, and on the principles of professional self regulation see Gunning & English, 1993; Mulkay, 1997; and Johnson, 1998.)

In this chapter, I will deal solely with that part of the HFE Act and its administration that is concerned with the statutory regulation of research and particularly with the application of research results to clinical practice: technology transfer or *therapeutic research*.

The research licensing system

The HFE Act functions to control research involving human embryos through a system of licensing. Without a license it is illegal to create, manipulate, store or use human embryos in vitro for research purposes. Licenses are issued by the HFEA upon receipt of a research application that satisfies a number of criteria legally specified in the HFE Act itself, as well as conforming to a Code of Practice which is issued and updated regularly by the HFEA (HFEA, 1998 and http://www.hfea.gov.uk/frame.htm). Each research project requires a separate application. Each application must have been approved in advance by a properly constituted local ethical committee. All applications are sent out by the HFEA for peer review.

There are relatively few prohibitions within the HFE Act that specify particular research activities and for which the HFEA does not have legal authority to issue a license. Those research activities which cannot be licensed are:

(i)   keeping or using a human embryo in vitro after the appearance of the primitive streak or after 14 days in vitro, whichever is the earlier;

(ii) placing an embryo in a non-human animal;

(iii) replacing a nucleus of a cell of an embryo with a nucleus taken from the cell of another person, another embryo, or a subsequent development of an embryo such as an embryonic cell line. This prohibits cloning by nuclear transfer to an embryonic cell but not to an oocyte - the "Dolly" technique (see later; Wilmut, Schnieke, McWhir & Campbell, 1997);

(iv) altering the genetic structure of any cell while it forms part of an embryo;

(v)   the mixing of gametes from different species, other than of a hamster egg with human sperm for the purposes of assessing the fertilizing capacity of the sperm, after which any fertilized egg resulting must be destroyed by the 2-cell stage.

In addition, a license cannot be granted unless the HFEA is satisfied that the use of human embryos is essential for the purposes of the research.

Otherwise, HFEA may grant licenses for research projects as long as they are likely to promote advances in the treatment of infertility, increase knowledge about the causes of congenital disease or miscarriages, develop more effective techniques of contraception, and/or develop methods for detecting the presence of gene or chromosome abnormalities in embryos before implantation. These are fairly broad and permissive categories of research objective. However, within this broad framework, the HFEA has stated that it will not license research projects involving embryo splitting with the intention of increasing the number of embryos for transfer, nor those involving replacement of an oocyte's chromosomes with a somatic nucleus ("Dolly" cloning). Either of these decisions could be amended by executive decision of the HFEA without recourse to legislation. The HFEA has also concluded that the broad categories above are insufficiently broad to cover research into the production of human cell lines or embryonic organs in vitro, for possible development of cell therapeutic uses. Further legislation may be required therefore for such research to become licensable.

In considering whether to issue a license, the HFEA will need to be reassured that there is appropriate patient information and available counseling and that patient written consent to the use of their gametes and/or embryos in research is valid and informed. It will also require evidence of the method to be used to terminate embryonic development, and of the procedure which will ensure that embryos do not continue to develop after fourteen days or (if earlier) the appearance of the primitive streak.

This approach to legislation is fundamentally flexible (see Johnson, 1998, for discussion). It is broadly capable of responding to changes in knowledge, social attitudes, and ethical thinking without recourse to primary legislation. It is also not such a hostage to fortune as might occur when precisely worded legislative prohibitions are rendered irrelevant by novel technological approaches (see Johnson 1997 for a more detailed discussion of this sort of problem).

This regulatory approach embodies two underlying assumptions:

(i) that licensing can be entrusted responsibly by Parliament (the democratically elected law makers) to a non-elected body of people (The HFEA) acting as a statutory body on Parliament's behalf. Appointment to membership of this body requires acceptance of the law being administered by the HFEA and collective responsibility for all decisions of the HFEA. Thus, whilst individual members may in discussion privately disagree with one another on specific issues, once a decision is made collectively it must be supported publicly by all members, given the statutory responsibilities of the HFEA. Checks on the activities of the HFEA include: the statutory law itself, the courts (through which its decisions and interpretations of the HFE Act can and have been challenged), the fact that its membership is controlled by Parliament through the Government, the fact that annual reports must be laid before Parliament, and the fact that the HFEA is answerable ultimately to Parliament and must respond to its demands.

(ii) a largely pragmatic or ethically consequentialist view that any issue is likely to be complex and to be made up of a balance of conflicting advantages and disadvantages. To discount the possibility of gaining advantages by an excess of specific prohibitions is not, therefore, in Society's best long term interests. In discussing the legislation, the UK Parliament was convinced that research involving human embryos or gametes in the process of fertilization could in certain circumstances be for

Society's good, and so approved broadly enabling legislation accordingly.

How does the licensing system regulate therapeutic research?

Under the HFE Act, licenses may be issued for research or for treatment, but not specifically for clinical trials of, for example, new technologies: therapeutic research. This is unhelpful and many consider that it represents a weakness in the HFE Act. However, this potential weakness can be overcome adequately within the flexible framework of the Act.

It is a standard condition of *all* licenses that where the clinic proposes to introduce *any* new activities or treatment services not specified in its existing license(s), these new activities or treatment services may not be commenced until the HFEA has been notified, has considered whether a new license may be needed, and, should this be so, an application has been made to and granted by the HFEA for a license relating to the new activities.

Thus, if clinics wishing to use a technique are uncertain as to whether it is "new" and therefore requires a license, they first enquire of the HFEA which makes a judgement after consulting both internally and externally. Technologies that have come into the category of "new" include, for example, laser-assisted zona hatching, use of the hypo-osmotic swelling (HOS) test on spermatozoa, use of spermatids in ICSI, and use of cryopreserved oocytes therapeutically. None of these techniques could be used in the UK unless an application for a license to use them has been approved.

If a technique is used without either enquiry or license application and the HFEA considers subsequently the technique to be new, the clinic is considered in breach of its license (if it has one for other purposes) or, less likely, to have performed a licensable technique illegally. Sanctions of various sorts can be applied locally, and information as to the need for a license disseminated generally to all clinics.

If the HFEA decides to license use of the new technology, it does so by issuing a license to treatment, but this license may impose such conditions as render it effectively a properly controlled and safe trial. In general therefore the criteria applied when granting a license for treatment by a therapeutic clinical research procedure will be much stricter than those imposed when granting a license for an established clinical treatment. Thus, the HFEA can control the introduction and dissemination of new techniques fairly robustly.

What is required for a new technique to be licensed for use therapeutically?

As was indicated in the previous section, although the HFEA cannot issue licenses for clinical trials *per se*, it effectively controls this process by attaching additional conditions to treatment licenses. These conditions are of three broad types.

First, no treatment license will be issued unless a clinic has demonstrated an adequate basis for proceeding to novel treatment. The criteria expected are no less than any responsible clinician would require to convince a properly constituted ethical or peer review committee, or indeed to convince an informed patient, that use of such a novel procedure was reasonably safe, efficacious and in the patient's best interests. These criteria would include a summary of the evidence from relevant work on animals, including data where appropriate, a reference list and copies of key references. This evidence would address the efficacy and reliability of the technique and any potential adverse effects. There must also be a summary of the evidence from research on human gametes or embryos (*without* replacement), including data where appropriate, a reference list and copies of key references. This evidence will use surrogate markers of developmental potential and normality such as appearance, developmental rates, damage rates, and genetic, cytological or biochemical analyses to address issues of safety and efficacy. If this evidence comes from the applying clinic, that clinic will of course previously have held a research license, one of the strengths of the UK system of allowing licensed research on human embryos to enhance the safety of therapeutic research. Finally, epidemiological data may be available for new treatments performed outside of the licensing area of the UK, and these will need to be properly presented with large enough numbers not to be simply anecdotal and with clear evidence that side effects have been sought and analyzed. Such reports will need to be validated by, for example, evidence of peer review. There is, however, no *requirement* for there to be data from embryo transfers for a new technique to be licensed. There is thus no requirement for UK scientists to go abroad to experiment in less regulated countries. It is accepted by the HFEA that research without transfer can only tell you so much and there comes a point at which the further step of transfer must be considered. It is the obligations surrounding the taking of this further step that must be clearly understood and addressed by applicant clinics.

Second, clinics must demonstrate competence to perform the novel therapeutic technique. In general, clinics will only apply for a license for a new technique when they already have licenses for standard techniques e.g.

IVF-ET, ICSI, PGD or DI. Technically they apply to "vary" their license to include the new technique. It is unlikely that clinics would be granted licenses for new techniques until they have demonstrated competence at standard techniques. In the UK, the granting of a license to perform ICSI requires that potential ICSI operatives and their equipment are all inspected and they are observed undertaking procedures. For use of spermatids in ICSI, it would be essential to demonstrate that the clinic could recognize a spermatid and discriminate it reliably from a Sertoli cell or lymphocyte. Another advantage of the ability of UK clinics to undertake licensed research on human embryos is that their competence to then move to therapy is likely to be greater than that in clinics which are simply adopting new clinical procedures derived from research performed elsewhere.

Third, the applying clinic would need to specify the patient population for the initial treatment cycles, including numbers and categories of patient, together with a justification for these based on evidence. For example, for novel zona hatching techniques the patient profile and treatment history may be relevant: there might be concern if the technique was to be applied to all patients as this might increase the risk of multiple pregnancies. The patient information must be submitted, together with details of how it will be used. It would need to be comprehensible and complete, and independent counseling should be offered. The consent form for the new treatment must be submitted. The clinic, if a license was granted, might be asked to report back to the HFEA on a case by case basis or after a defined number of treatment attempts or outcomes.

In applying these criteria to license applications from clinics for permission to perform new therapeutic treatments, the HFEA and its referees will be looking for evidence that the applicant clinic has clearly understood the requirements of the Code of Practice that specify:

> Eggs or sperm which have been subjected to procedures which carry an actual or reasonable theoretical risk of harm to their developmental potential, and embryos created from them, should not be used for treatment. Treatment centers should satisfy the HFEA that sufficient scientific evidence is available to establish that any procedures used do not prejudice the developmental potential of the gametes or embryos.

and

> embryos which have themselves been subject to procedures which carry an actual or reasonable theoretical risk of harm to their developmental potential should not be used for treatment. Treatment centers should satisfy the HFEA

that sufficient scientific evidence is available to establish that any procedures used do not prejudice the developmental potential of the embryos.

and

Gametes or embryos which have been exposed to a material risk of contamination which might cause harm to recipients or to any resulting children should not be used for treatment. If there is any doubt, centers should seek expert advice.

How is a license then issued, varied or refused?

The accumulated evidence with the application will usually be sent to independent referees in confidence for comments according to established criteria. These include consideration of legal constraints, ethical considerations and medico-scientific knowledge and judgement. The application then passes with these comments to a licensing committee of a sub-group of members of the HFEA. The committee decides whether or not to grant a license. It may ask the applying clinic for more evidence or information and defer a decision. It can also refer any matters to one or more of its specialist working groups, such as the Ethics Committee or the Working Group for consideration of New Reproductive Technologies. These working groups are made up of HFEA members plus coopted experts. If the licensing committee issues a license it will impose conditions on the use of the license which may include, *inter alia*, limits on the type or numbers of patients, changes to the patient information or consent form or to clinical protocols, report back procedures, etc. It may also make recommendations to the clinic about the conduct of the new therapy: these are usually intended to be helpful to the clinic, based as they are on the collective experience of the HFEA members and its advisers. Subsequently, at its annual inspection, these conditions and recommendations will all be raised with the clinic to establish compliance. If the license is refused, the reasons are given.

Conclusions

Few would say that the licensing system in the UK is perfect. However, given that regulation of research and therapy involving human embryos in vitro seems to be becoming an inevitable feature of most Societies (Johnson, 1998), the general principles underlying regulation by the HFE Act seem to be broadly constructive and have lead to workable practices. It is arguable that of the proposed seven criteria suggested for maximal effectiveness of a statutory regulatory body (Johnson, 1998), criteria iv, vi, and vii are of particular relevance for therapeutic research.

Criterion (vi) suggests that the regulatory body should function in a way that allows imaginative scientists, doctors and others to make the case for change and should enable them to collect the evidence required to make that case convincingly. This criterion is undoubtedly fulfilled, as is hopefully made clear in this article.

However, criterion (iv) suggests that the regulatory body should not stray unduly from regulation by underlying principles into the regulation of professional practice and standards which is more properly the province of professional self regulating bodies which should be encouraged to undertake this role and not to feel disempowered by legislation. It is arguable that in its response to applications for licenses to apply new therapeutic technologies the HFEA is too prescriptive, refusing or delaying applications unreasonably, or imposing conditions and making recommendations that hamper clinicians. Indeed, the HFEA has been accused by clinicians and patients of precisely this in respect of the introduction of new technologies such as ICSI with round spermatids and use of frozen oocytes. However, critics would need to make the case that the HFEA has indeed been presented with all the evidence quite reasonably required of them, or has been informed clearly and unambiguously of what further evidence is needed. If they can do this, then the HFEA would stand indicted of breaching this criterion. Furthermore, there is little evidence in respect of therapeutic research and innovation that the HFEA is out of step with professional bodies or patient organizations in its views. Indeed it would be surprising if it were, given that many members of such bodies are represented on the HFEA and its advisory panels.

Criterion (vii) suggests that the regulatory body should offer leadership in the debate and thinking about ART, including the introduction of new therapeutic techniques, through consultation, education and the use of an involving process of working that draws all sections of society into its activities as far as is possible. The HFEA certainly meets this criterion in respect of its use of advisers from a range of fields and in its many consultation documents.

A regulatory body such as the HFEA has the difficult task of balancing multiple interests in respect of the introduction of new reproductive technologies. It must address the special status of the human embryo in vitro respectfully, facilitate the creativity of scientists and doctors that leads to innovation and advance, meet the reasonable (and often sadly the desperately unreasonable) expectations of the infertile patients whilst attempting to maximize both their autonomy and the safety of their treatment, protect the interests of children to be born, ensure public safety, and respect social ethic, and it must do all this in a way which conforms with the law and through actions for which it is answerable to Parliament and the Courts. This is a demanding role.

References

Gunning, J. & English, V. (1993) *Human in vitro Fertilization: A Case Study in the Regulation of Medical Innovation*. Dartmouth Press.

HFEA (1990) Human Fertilisation and Embryology Act , HMSO, London.

HFEA (1998) Human Fertilisation and Embryology Authority, Code of Practice. 4th Edition, Paxton House, 30 Artillery Lane, London E1 7LS.

Johnson, M.H. (1997) 'Cloning Humans?' *BioEssays* vol. 19, pp. 737-739.

Johnson, M.H. (1998) 'Should the use of Assisted Reproduction Techniques be Deregulated?' *Human Reproduction* vol. 13, pp. 1769-1776.

Mulkay, M. (1997) *The Embryo Research Debate: Science and the Politics of Reproduction*. Cambridge University Press, Cambridge.

Wilmut, I., Schnieke, A.E., McWhir, A.J., and Campbell, K.H.S. (1997) 'Viable offspring derived from fetal and adult mammalian cells'. *Nature* vol. 385, pp. 810-812.

13 The Role of Ethics Committees in Framing Legislation on Assisted Reproduction and Embryo Research

LINDA NIELSEN

Denmark

In April 1984 the Danish Minister of the Interior established a committee to investigate the ethical problems connected with genetic engineering, in vitro fertilization, artificial insemination and prenatal diagnosis. In the Committee's report, "The Price of Progress" the establishment of an ethics council for the health system was recommended. In 1987 the Danish Parliament adopted a bill to set up the Danish Council of Ethics.[1] The role of the Danish Council of Ethics is to examine biomedical and ethical questions and to produce proposals for legislation. Apart from advising the Parliament and the health service authorities on ethical issues, the Council's mandate is to "keep the public up to date on developments and its work and to assume the initiative of making ethical questions the subject of debate among the public". The Council makes annual reports both in Danish and in English.

When appointing members the Minister of Health has to consider the appointees publicly substantiated knowledge of the ethical, cultural and social questions of importance to the work of the Council. Nine members are appointed by a committee appointed by Parliament and these nine members are made up, politically, in the same proportions as Parliament. However, the members appointed by Parliament must not be Members of Parliament, or members of Municipal or County councils. When the committee cannot agree on an appointment, the majority of the committee is used to decide on the appointment. Council appointments must ensure equal presentation of men and women – there may be only be one more of one sex than of the other. The chairman is appointed by the Minister of

Health from among the appointees on the recommendation of the parliamentary committee. The members and chairman are appointed for a term of three years. Reappointment may take place once. The parliamentary committee is required to follow the work of the Council of Ethics by means of joint meetings. Furthermore, the committee can ask the Council of Ethics to deal with specified subjects within the Councils terms of reference. The Council of Ethics shall, according to the Act, have a permanent secretariat, the staff of which shall be employed and dismissed by the Minister of Health on the recommendation of the chairman of the Council. The necessary funds for the work of the Council are granted in annual budgets.

At the same time as the beginning of the work of the Danish Council of Ethics, a temporary prohibition concerning embryo research was laid down in the law. The legislation provided that a number of specific matters should be reviewed and that the legislative proposals should be laid before Parliament in the session 1989-90 at the latest.

This "interim" approach to regulation is based on the view that the issues at stake were of such importance that a legal vacuum was quite inappropriate and the law was enacted to provide what, in effect, amounted to a moratorium on embryo research and a restriction on the uses of assisted conception until the Danish Council of Ethics had the opportunity to address the social, legal and ethical questions which it believed these developments disclosed. The Danish Council of Ethics had the ethical problems regarding assisted reproduction and embryo research on the agenda in 1989. The Council produced background and briefing papers, held public meetings and published a book of proceedings in order to inform and stimulate public debate. Specific interest groups and public and private institutions were asked to comment before the Council presented its report.[2]

The Council was charged by the legislation to proceed on the basis that human life begins at the time of conception. The intention of this provision was later interpreted by the Minister of the Interior in responding to a question from the parliamentary committee responsible for the Ethics Council as not to give a definition of human life and its inception. The intent with the formulation has been to:

> establish that the Council of Ethics ought to work from the basis that it is not ethically or legally an argument for unlimited freedom of action toward the human ovum that this is not human life, or expressed the other way round, that from the moment of conception on, a situation exists where it is ethically and legally necessary to consider and perhaps introduce particular limitations in the freedom of action.

The Act did not prevent later legislation accepting embryo research.

The 1992 Act

In 1991 a draft Danish bill was published and the resulting legislation[3] came into force in October 1992 with a statutory obligation to undertake review and revision if necessary by 1995-96. The Act deals with Ethics Review Committees and treatment of biomedical research projects. It includes regulation as to research on embryos and donation and cryopreservation of human eggs and embryos.

The 1992 Act sanctioned embryo research up to 14 days after fertilization. The proviso is that the object of the research, sanctioned by a regional as well as the central committee must be the improvement of techniques of in vitro fertilization with a view to promoting pregnancy. Removing and fertilizing eggs or embryos for any other purpose was prohibited. The legal motives (explanatory memorandum) appended to the bill make it clear that the main reason for accepting research but restricting it in this way is that IVF is a recognized treatment and that research is accepted internationally as an integrated part of the development of treatment. Prohibiting all research would mean consciously offering less optimal treatment than possible.

The 1992 legislation provided that any biomedical research project which includes research on living human individuals, human gametes which are intended for use in fertilization, fertilized human eggs, pre-embryos or embryos shall be reported to regional ethics committees. There are presently seven such committees, established according to local government boundaries and they comprise 9 or 11 members, three of whom are nominated by the state authorized scientific committee. A central ethics committee is established by the Minister of Research, who appoints two members. In addition, two members are appointed by the Minister of Health and two members are appointed by each of the regional committees. The central and regional committees are charged to oversee and where appropriate to approve research.

1995 Report from the Danish Council of Ethics

The Danish Council of Ethics took up the topic of assisted reproduction in 1995 with the intention of forming part of the basis for work on legislative policy in the field in connection with the 1995-96 revision of the Danish Act on the Scientific and Ethical Committee System, which contains some regulations on assisted reproduction. The report was first published in draft form to provide a debate outline for the specific occasion of the Council of Ethics' debate day on September 5, 1995. Against the background of discussions on the debate day and the public debate generally fuelled by the draft report, the Council revised this draft and presented a report in its final form later in 1995.

In the 1994 report[4] there was consensus among the Council on a number of general points. There was agreement on the need to consolidate research into the origins of infertility and into curative treatment aimed at eliminating the causes of infertility. Moreover, there was a broad consensus that assisted reproduction is such a sensitive and important area as to warrant public supervision and monitoring of developments in the field. The Council's members were united in recommending overall regulation of the field, which includes placing approval procedures for new forms of treatment on a statutory footing. Similarly the Council's members agreed that it is of the utmost importance to provide increased guidance and counseling for couples seeking treatment, both prior to commencing treatment and during the treatments. At the same time it is important even at an early stage to inform them about the available alternatives to assisted reproduction, e.g. adoption. In this connection an unanimous Councils also wished to recommend that the rules governing adoption and in vitro fertilization be aligned with regard to prerequisites and finance. There was further agreement amongst the Council that there should be a mandatory upper age limit for women being treated for infertility, a ceiling to be applied both in the public hospital sector and at the private clinics. The justification for this age cut-off is primarily out of consideration for the child-to-be, who wherever possible should be given normal conditions under which to grow up. There was further agreement within the Council that artificial insemination with partner's sperm and the freezing of sperm are techniques that do not give rise to any ethical misgivings.

Finally there was agreement among the Council that the cloning of fertilized eggs with a view to producing genetically identical human beings, the use of eggs from aborted fetuses, the transplantation of ovaries and the freezing of unfertilized eggs must be banned in Denmark.

The disagreement on the Council concerned whether to impose additional limitations on the access to infertility treatment and on the range of techniques that can be used in treatment. A majority of Council members considered that assisted reproduction in which fertilization takes place outside the woman's body represents a "technologization" and a reification of the reproductive process. It was the view of these members that such techniques involve changes in our view of human life and of reproduction itself, changes which appear to affect social and cultural development in an unwished-for direction. A minority on the Council felt, in opposition to the majority, that the regulation of assisted reproduction should be confined to its present level. These members did not think that the techniques available in Denmark at the time produced sufficient ethical misgivings to justify being banned. On the contrary, the minority felt that the couples seeking treatment see their infertility as a great strain and that the help motive therefore dictates that treatment should be made available. Speaking quite generally, these members also felt that there is a vigorous tradition of mutual tolerance in Denmark and an extensive degree of respect for the individual's right of self-determination. The question of whether or not the various techniques are ethically acceptable should therefore be left up to those who would be involved in the treatment.

The Council of Ethics' report contains a discussion of a further three questions central to the debate on assisted reproduction. First, the question of abolishing the current practice whereby both egg and sperm donors are assured anonymity. Next, the question of whether single women and women living in lesbian relationships are to have access to assisted reproduction. Finally, the question of whether infertility treatment should still take place in the publicly funded health service. A majority on the Council of Ethics felt that donor anonymity ought to be rescinded for future donors. This outlook is primarily justified by consideration for the child. With regard to the question of access to assisted reproduction services for single status persons and lesbian women a majority of the Council of Ethics was in favor of no ban on assisted reproduction being introduced for these groups of women. Finally, the Council of Ethics was of the overall opinion that the question of whether to offer infertility treatment in the public health service should be seen in correlation with the broader issue of how to prioritize the resources of the health sector. A majority of the Council members still feel that infertility treatment should be offered in the public health sector.

The 1997 Act

In 1997 the Act on assisted reproduction was amended again. The current legislation thus covers assisted reproduction where doctors are involved.[5] The 1997 Act stipulates – as something new compared to the 1992 Act – in Article 3, that artificial reproduction may only be offered to women who are married or cohabiting with a man. A written consent from the woman and her husband or partner is needed. The provision in Article 3 was not in the original bill but was introduced in Parliament during the negotiations and was accepted with a very narrow difference in votes for and against. Moreover, artificial reproduction may now only take place in cases where the woman who is to give birth to the child in no older than 45 years.

According to the 1997 Act fertilized and unfertilized eggs may be cryopreserved up to two years, after which period they are to be destroyed. In the case of the man or the woman's death or in case of separation or divorce between the parties or the end of cohabitation, the cryopreserved fertilized eggs are to be destroyed. The "spouse" or "cohabitant" cryopreserved and fertilized eggs are also to be destroyed in the case of the woman's death. In practice cryopreservation of embryos is being done whereas the safe and reliable cryopreservation of unfertilized human eggs is not yet possible.

The 1997 Act only contains a few provisions dealing with donor insemination. It is expressly stated that the spouse's or cohabitant's cryopreserved semen is to be destroyed in the case of the man's death. Moreover, it is emphasized, that the Minister of Health is authorized to make further administrative regulations regarding storing, donation and use of donor sperm. According to these administrative regulations donor insemination is to be undertaken anonymously. Donation of human eggs is accepted when these are unfertilized. Such donation with the purpose of achieving a pregnancy with another woman is only permissible where eggs are taken as part of an IVF treatment of the donating woman. Artificial reproduction with an egg donated by another woman may not take place if the donating woman's identity is known beforehand by the receiving couple and likewise the receiving couple cannot beforehand decide the identity of the donor.

Donation of embryos – fertilized human eggs – is banned. Artificial reproduction may not be undertaken unless the egg cell derives from the women who gives birth to the child or the semen derives from her partner.

Surrogacy is explicitly banned when it is performed in connection with artificial reproduction. Artificial reproduction may not take place even when an agreement between the surrogate mother and another woman (the prospective mother) exists.

It is not admissible to bring unfertilized or fertilized human eggs which have been obtained in Denmark, with the aim of reproduction or research, to another country and it is not permissible to sell, procure sale or in other ways to contribute to the sale of unfertilized or fertilized human eggs.

As something new, the 1997 Act stipulates that sex selection of sperm or fertilized eggs before implantation is banned unless this happens with the aim of preventing a sex-linked hereditary disease. The development of a fertilized egg into a human individual may not take place outside a woman's womb and the use of immature eggs or ovaries from aborted fetuses or deceased women may not take place. Transplantation of ovaries to another woman with the aim of treating infertility may not take place. Artificial reproduction may not be undertaken unless it is performed with the aim of uniting an unchanged (unmodified) oocyte with genetically unchanged (unmodified) sperm.

Finally the 1997 Act contains the same prohibitions as the 1991 Act regarding embryo research, cloning, and hybrids.

Norway

In Norway Act No. 68 of 12 June 1987, concerning artificial fertilization establishes that this may be carried out only in institutions specially approved for the purpose by the Ministry of Social Affairs. The freezing of unfertilized eggs is prohibited. Only those establishments which are authorized to carry out artificial fertilization may freeze or store sperm or fertilized eggs. The latter may be utilized only for implantation and may not be preserved for more than twelve months. Research on fertilized eggs is forbidden.

Artificial fertilization is restricted to the treatment of married women.

Generally IVF may only take place if the woman or her husband of partner is infertile or if they are, for reasons unknown, infertile as a couple. However, IVF may also be used in cases of serious hereditary disease. The decision to undertake treatment with a view to artificial reproduction has to be made by a physician. The decision is to be based on a medical and psycho-social assessment of the couple. The couple must be given information about the treatment and the medical and legal consequences it may have.

Assisted reproduction treatment may be carried out only in married women or women living in a stable partnership with a man. According to the explanatory memorandum, a certain stability is necessary; approximately three to five years. The involvement of medical science in the creation of human life and the allocation of technical, medical and economic resources from society is seen as an opportunity to take into account the interest of the child. While the creation of one-parent families cannot be averted, the deliberate use of assisted conception services in such circumstances is seen to offend against the rights of the individual child who will result. Before treatment is embarked upon, written consent has to be obtained from the woman and her husband or partner. The physician providing treatment must ensure that the consent is still valid at the start of the treatment.

Sperm may only be imported with permission from the Norwegian Health Board

Donor insemination may be carried out only when the husband is infertile or if he himself suffers from or is the carrier of a serious hereditary disease or, in special cases, where the woman is the carrier of a recessive gene of which the man is also a carrier. The physician providing the treatment shall select a suitable sperm donor. In Norway the identity of the donor is to be kept secret. A sperm donor shall not be given information regarding the identity of the couple or the child. The treatment of sperm before implantation with a view to determining the sex of the child is allowed only if the woman is the carrier of a serious sex-linked hereditary disease.

IVF may be carried out only with the gametes of the couples themselves – neither donor sperm nor donor eggs may be used in conjunction with IVF. The embryo may be used only for implantation in the woman from whom the eggs originate. The reason for banning egg donation is primarily in the interest of the child as it is argued that egg donation would deprive the child of a link which is fundamental to its identity. Moreover, it has been emphasized that egg donation breaks the natural link between uterus and egg and makes it possible to manipulate the identity of the mother. Egg donation would open up a whole new series of problems concerning the identity and the roots of the child. Finally the ethical considerations are linked to the risk of manipulating the identity of the mother and the risk of selection and commercialization. The risk is considered to outweigh the right of personal freedom and autonomy of the couples wishing for a child.

Regarding paternity, Norwegian legislation considers the spouse or cohabitant as legal father in cases where he has consented to donor insemination unless it is likely that the child is a fruit of the donor insemination. The donor cannot be considered as the legal father by a court decision and he is secured anonymity – and cannot obtain information about the identity of the child or the couple. In 1997 Norway introduced the right for a man who considered himself the father of a child to take legal proceedings concerning paternity until the child is three years of age. The court may grant an exemption.

New provisions concerning maternity have been introduced in the 1997 legislation on children and parents. It is emphasized that even if Norway does not allow egg donation, other countries do, and thus a provision states that the woman giving birth to the child is to be considered the child's legal mother. The reasoning is that the woman has carried the child through pregnancy and has obtained a special emotional attachment to it. Moreover, equality arguments relating to sperm donation have been mentioned. These arguments are seen as overriding the fact that the egg donor is the genetic mother of the child. At the same time a provision was introduced stating that an agreement to give birth to a child for another woman is not legally binding. Thus a surrogate contract will be invalid according to Norwegian legislation.

In Norway embryo research is not allowed but somatic gene therapy has specifically come under legislation. Future use of somatic gene therapy is conditional on aiming at the treatment of serious disease and each new treatment has to be approved by the Social Department. Germ line gene therapy is not allowed. The danger of altering the human species has been emphasized in the explanatory memorandum.

The choice of a particular sex is prohibited unless specific sex-dependent grave diseases justify it.

Sweden

According to Law No. 1140 of 20 December 1984 on donor insemination, this may only take place on the condition that the woman is married or cohabits with a man under marriage like conditions. Donor insemination may only take place in a public hospital under the supervision of a physician qualified in obstetrics and gynecology. The physician shall determine if it is appropriate that insemination take place taking into consideration the medical, psychological and social circumstances of the couple. Insemination may take place only if it is probable that the child resulting therefrom will be brought up under favorable conditions. The physician shall select an appropriate sperm donor.

The most radical aspect of this law is the section relating to information about the donor. Sweden was the first country in the world to enact legislation concerned with the practice of donor insemination. The 1984 Act decrees that the child should have the right to obtain identifying information about the donor, when the child has reached sufficient maturity. The argument has relied upon concerns for the welfare and interests of the child. It is considered a basic right of a child to know its origin. Without it the child will be deprived of the possibility of having a true conception of him- or herself. The social authorities are obliged, at the request of the child to assist in procuring such information. The child's right is not offset by a right for the donor to know the child's identity.

According to the explanatory memorandum the regulation has taken on board the experience gained from adoption, where children from studies are known to benefit from receiving information about their genetic origin, providing that the information comes from people who like them and respect their wish. Mention is also made of the fact that secrecy entraps the parents in a lifelong lie. In terms of logistics the child can look up the social services committee and have a talk with a staff member in the same way as happened in the case of an adopted child. The staff member can then disclose information about the donor. If the child wishes to have contact with the donor, this takes place through the hospital where the insemination was carried out. The social services officer is of assistance in trying to trace the donor and may even contact him.

The net effect of the change of attitude to donor anonymity represented in the law was, firstly, to reduce the number of donors. The demand has also since declined with the possibility of ICSI to address the problems of male infertility. More recently the number of donors has increased again. At the same time there has been a change in the type of donor available; older married men rather than younger single men are offering themselves as donors. In fact, it has been documented in an article from 1995 that while there was a temporary decline in the number of donors in some clinics, this decline has now been reversed. It is suggested in the article that the possibility of future contact by genetic offspring has not had the negative impact on the availability of donors predicted. There is not yet any experience published about the extent and the psychological "success or failure" regarding contact between the child and the donor father.

According to Law No. 711 of 14 June 1988 on fertilization outside the human body, this may only be carried out in a general hospital, unless the authorization of the National Board of Health and Welfare is obtained. An egg which has been fertilized outside the body of a woman may not be introduced into her body unless the woman is married or living in a state of cohabitation and the egg is the woman's own and has been fertilized with the sperm of her husband or cohabitant.

In Sweden there is a licensing system with regard to the clinics performing assisted reproduction. Treatment may not be administered anywhere other than at public hospitals without the permission of the National Board of Health and Welfare.

Donor insemination and IVF are restricted to married couples or those living together in a permanent relationship – more than two years. The husband or the partner must furnish written consent for the treatment.

Freezing of surplus embryos is allowed for up to one year with the couple's consent. The National Board of Health may allow a more prolonged time span if there are 'marked reasons' for it. Only establishments which are authorized to carry out artificial fertilization may freeze or store sperm or fertilized eggs. The latter may be utilized only for implantation in women.

The use of donated gametes in the context of IVF or the donation of surplus embryos to another couple is forbidden in Swedish law. The reasoning is that donor insemination in itself constitutes a deviation from the natural process. Where the donation of ova is concerned, it is considered that the use of eggs from a third party is contrary to the human biological process. Moreover, considerations concerning the wellbeing of the future child have been emphasized. There has been thought given in Sweden to changing this but it has not been done so far.

In Sweden embryo research is not permitted beyond 14 days after fertilization. A fertilized egg which has been subject to research must be destroyed without delay after the expiry of two weeks. If a fertilized egg has been subjected to research, it must not be introduced into a woman's body. The law is silent on the creation of embryos for research.

Germ line gene therapy is prohibited in the Swedish legislation and research must not have the intention of developing methods of creating genetic effects which can be hereditary.

The role played by ethics committees with regard to legislation

The debate initiated by the Danish Council of Ethics has influenced the legislation and especially the arguments underlying proposals and legislation. As the Danish Council of Ethics in their reports – most radically in the 1989 report but also in the 1995 report – have different opinions on a number of subjects, including majority and minority views, you cannot say that the legislation has followed the Council's advice. What you can say is that the arguments underlying the different approaches by members of the Council of Ethics have influenced the arguments introduced before Parliament. This is reflected in the widespread debate and remarks made in the Danish Parliament and published in the "Folketingets forhandlinger".

The (personal) arguments are of special interest. As the area of assisted reproduction has been considered such a personal and sensitive area, members of Parliament have not – as is usual – been bound by the approach taken by their political party but have expressly been free to give their own personal opinion.

Thus I think it is fair to say that the work of the Danish Council of Ethics is influential on the debate and the underlying arguments but not necessarily on the legislative result, which is natural, as members of Parliament differ as much in opinions and approaches as do the members of the Council of Ethics.

In this respect it is of importance that the Danish Council of Ethics in their report both say when a majority is of a special opinion and when a minority has a different opinion but also places the names of how different people voted for different approaches in the report. This way each and every member of the Council has to give their personal opinion and the press and the politicians are afterwards very interested in the opinion of each member.

As chairman of the Council it was my effort to try to make room for different opinions and approaches and to make the presentation of them clear. It was not, however, my role to try to achieve a consensus when there was not one present. This is contrary to the working of many other governmental committees but is based on the fact that the primary task of the Council is to produce arguments for public debate and political decision making and these arguments, in my opinion, are best presented in their clear forms. Then the politicians can choose between the arguments and the opinions and make political decisions.

In Norway and Sweden some of these remarks and considerations will also be relevant but the tradition has to a further extent in Norway and Sweden, rather than in Denmark, been to have reports made by governmental committees.

Notes

1   Act No. 353 of June 3rd 1987 on the Establishment of an ethical council and the Regulation of Certain Forms of Biomedical Experiments.
2   The Danish Council of Ethics' Second Annual Report, 1989; Protection of Human Gametes, Fertilized Ova, Embryos and Fetuses, 1990.
3   Act No 503 of June 24 1992.
4   Published in the Danish Council of Ethics Annual Report, 1995.
5   Act No 480 June 10 1997 on artificial fertilization in connection with medical treatment, diagnosis and research.

14 The Hungarian Legislative Approach to Assisted Procreation: An Attempt at Transparency?

JUDIT SÁNDOR

Ten years ago Hungarian society underwent a profound economic and political change. Pluralist society, multi-party system and foundations for the market economy had been developed in a relatively short period of the political-economic transition. For the Hungarian doctors the year of 1989 meant not only the dawn of the new political regime but it was regarded also as the starting point of assisted procreation, since the first in vitro baby was born "together with the democracy" in 1989. Slowly the entire scope of reproductive services were practiced, even including ICSI and surrogacy.[1] Still until 1997 there was no comprehensive regulation on assisted procreation.

After a long silence, in 1997 a new reproduction regulation developed in Hungary, though without a significant public debate and without previously existing reproductive policy. Despite of all the difficulties in 1997 the Hungarian Parliament voted for the Act that focused mainly on the needs of infertile couples.

Assisted procreation, although practiced in Hungary for about 10 years, received little public attention and even less legal and ethical control before 1997. The first successful GIFT was made in 1987 in Pecs (in the southern part of Hungary), and shortly after that the first in vitro baby was born in 1989. Since then, in Hungary numerous private and public medical centers provide biomedical assistance for infertile couples. In this process it has been very difficult to formulate a consistent view on such a controversial and not yet debated issue as assisted procreation.

Reproductive regulation was not an isolated attempt to create transparency in the health care sector. It was a part of a broader regulative reform initiated by the Hungarian Ministry for Welfare. The reform started after some deliberation in 1996 with the aim to provide a comprehensive Health Care Act. This reform was implicitly based on two principles. One was to stress the new, autonomy based doctor-patient relationship. The second aim was to cover the areas of new technologies and development of the national health care system. As a result of these efforts a new, comprehensive Act was produced by the participation of about 150 experts. This new Act, for the first time in the history of Hungarian medical law, gave priority to patients' rights. In December 1997 the Hungarian Parliament already adopted a new comprehensive Health Act that influenced the entire sphere of medical law. The new Health Care Act promoted the principle of patient autonomy and provided enforceable rights for the patients. This legislative manner was in sharp contrast to the previous regulative solution that imposed vague and unenforceable duties on the health care professionals. Emphasis on patient's rights was further underlined by the application of a concrete, instead of an abstract formulation of rights.

The Health legislation had been motivated also by political reasons since patients' rights were on the agenda of the Socialist-Liberal Governmental Coalition. In December 1997 the new Health Act (Act No CLIV) was adopted by the Parliament. In order to provide sufficient time for implementation and to draft additional Governmental decrees the Act came into force only in July, 1998. Between the adoption the Health Care Act and the promulgation of further health care decrees the election radically changed the political climate since after the election a new, Conservative-Christian coalition came to power. A new ministerial decree has come into force, as well. [30/1998 (VI.24.) NM.]

Although in the future some changes may be expected in the Health Act, nevertheless the trends toward a patients' rights oriented health care system seemed to become irreversible from the time of this codification.

It is still difficult to predict the potential effects of this Act and to assess the overall consequences of the new regulation. In the following paragraphs I will very briefly describe the main elements of the new Hungarian law.

Regulation on Assisted Procreation in Hungary has two levels at the moment: a chapter in the Parliamentary Act on health care and the Ministry decree: The 1997.CLIV. Parliamentary Act on Health Care Chapter IX. (Articles 165-187) can be considered as the main reproductive law that was specified in the 30/ 1998.(VI.24.). NM r. (decree of the Ministry of Welfare) "on extraordinary procedures of human reproduction, the treatment of embryos, gametes and their storage" developed the technical and medical requirements for the assisted reproductive services. The Ministry decree also encompasses extraordinary procedures of human reproduction, the treatment of embryos, gametes and their storage.

The 1997 Health Act includes a Chapter on assisted procreation providing main rules for access and the condition for the different forms of assisted procreation. The 1997. CLIV. Parliamentary Act on Health Care in Chapter IX. (Articles 165-187) regulates the "extraordinary treatments of human reproduction, research on human embryos and gametes" and also provides rules for sterilization. To find an appropriate title for this Chapter in the Health Act was already a challenging job for the drafting committee.

At the time when in 1996 the Hungarian Ministry of Welfare made the decision to initiate a comprehensive law-reform relatively little attention was paid to the problems of assisted procreation. Although eight in vitro centers had already been in operation (7 public and one private)[2] still the general public had a very little knowledge about the ethical and legal issues of these medical interventions.

Hungarian society is often described by sociologists as a child-loving society, even despite of the fact that statistical figures show low birth rates and relatively high abortion rates. In 1994 a survey[3] showed much stronger preference to live with children in Hungary than in other countries in the region. In another study that compared eight European countries with respect to the willingness to pay or assisted procreation or even to travel to foreign countries to obtain these services, Hungary seemed to demonstrate the highest attention and desire for these technologies.[4]

Basic features of the Hungarian Reproduction law

Although the Hungarian Health Act does not specifically mention the underlying principles of the reproductive provisions, nevertheless during the debates the following principles were crystallized:

a) Assisted procreation should be recognized as a substitution of natural procreation, therefore it is a form of palliative treatment (only for infertile couples).
b) Only spouses and heterosexual couples living in common law marriage (only one relationship) may request MAP.
c) All the procedure should be initiated by the written joint request of the couple. (In case of a request for the continuation of assisted

procreation by a widowed or divorced woman, a written statement in front of a notary is required).

d)   A special informed consent procedure need to be followed in the course of these treatments that includes the further perspectives and medical treatment that may become necessary in conjunction with the initiated treatment (e.g. embryo reduction).

e)   Strong preference should be given to personality rights (this effort seemed to be unsuccessful in some articles where a strong property law language was applied).

f)   There should be prohibition and elimination of commercialization of gamete and embryo donation.

The current Health Act, though regarded as relatively liberal, imposes some restrictions in assisted procreation, such as the use of gametes from a cadaver, using other than human gametes, creating an embryo for research purposes, implanting human embryos into animals, sex selection of embryos (except for genetic disease inherited only by one of the sexes), and implanting human embryos into human body after embryo research. In the case of using donated gametes, the donor of the gametes should be not older than 35 and not more than four offspring should be born by using the same donor's gametes.

Embryo transfer is limited to up to three embryos, except for women older than 35 who may request the transfer of 4 embryos and in some other cases when there is a strong medical indication for the transfer of 4 embryos (previous unsuccessful embryo transfer).

Most of the restrictions are based on pragmatic rather than ethical concerns while others reflect the minimal ethical consensus in Europe.

During the 1996-1997 legislative process even single women's access to reproduction services were discussed but during drafting of the Parliamentary Act it was rejected. A peculiarity of the Hungarian law is the formulation of a new reproductive right, the right to request the continuation of assisted procreation. This right was incorporated based on deliberation and analysis of some warning lessons drawn from other countries, (mainly by the French jurisdiction in which significant litigation[5] occurred due to the rejected claims of the widows to request for the continuation of the treatment if the fertilization had been already completed). This legal innovation in the Hungarian law was related to an indirect recognition of the inequality of the situation in women and men's in assisted procreation. While sperm donation is regarded to be more close to the process of natural coitus and does not have any risk, egg donation includes lengthy hormonal treatment, and egg aspiration itself is an invasive and often painful intervention with significant risks. Because of those risks, egg aspiration cannot be performed without any limitation. The Hungarian position therefore rejects the approach that considers the biopsy like egg aspiration to be identical to sperm donation from the aspect of medical law. Since hormonal treatment and subsequent egg aspiration is regarded as a more invasive form of medical intervention than sperm donation Hungarian law created a special right for widows and divorced women if they remained alone after the egg had been already fertilized. I am sure these solutions will be regarded benevolently by some pro-life activists, as well. So far there was no litigation in this respect, though in the future some controversies might be expected, especially concerning divorced women.

The Hungarian law has regard for the differences between the male and female contribution to assisted procreation treatment, nevertheless, in the case of divorced women the potential problems with respect to family law had not yet been elaborated through the lack of judicial cases.

In order to minimize litigation in this field, a legal guarantee was introduced to help to arrange this kind of debate. In the beginning of an assisted procreation treatment, the couple has to be notified about this legal arrangement and, if it seems undesirable to them, they may exclude this solution by their mutual written request at the beginning of the treatment and before the wife has started to undergo hormonal stimulation.

Nevertheless, the couple has to be notified about the legal possibility of continuation and they may exclude this option at the beginning of the treatment by means of a common written request.

Controlling and monitoring mechanism

The Human Reproduction Committee, the main controlling and licensing agency was created by the 1997 law.[6] Although the Committee exists *de jure* however, it does not yet operate. As a consequence the attempt towards transparency seems to be still incomplete. The Committee has still not started to function two years after the law created it.

Some confusion might be due to the 1997 Ministry decree that was adopted during drafting the Health Act. This Ministry decree[7] created a subordination by placing the Human Reproduction Commission under the Health Care and Science Council (Egészségügyi Tudományos Tanács) and, furthermore, prescribed roles and functions of the Human Reproduction Committee.

The technology based attitude could be easily recognized by the list of techniques in the Ministry decree. Techniques regulated by the 1997 Parliamentary Act and the 1998 Ministry decree: include *in vitro* fertilization and embryo transfer, IVF and embryo transfer with donated gametes, embryo transfer with donated embryos, GIFT (gamete intra-fallopian transfer), PROST (pro-nuclear stage transfer), ZIFT (zygote intra-fallopian transfer), TET (tubal embryo transfer), ICSI (intra-cytoplasmic sperm injection), ICSI-MESA (microsurgical sperm aspiration), ICSI-TESE (testicular sperm extraction), Assisted hatching (AH), embryo freezing, artificial insemination (AIH and AID), research on embryos.

The Law created general access to assisted procreation for couples who need these services based on exclusively medical grounds. A further condition is that assisted procreation techniques must follow a gradual approach ; that means, for example, that, if artificial insemination can be successful, doctors do not start with in vitro fertilization. The 1998 Ministerial decree further specified the medical indication of each of the MAP procedures.

Before starting the medical interventions the doctor has to provide full information about the MAP for the couple, both in written and in a verbal form. The content of information should be specific and should encompass the elements of the entire reproductive procedure.

The information provided should especially concern:

a) the medical indication of the procedure;
b) the nature of the intervention, the supplementary or the repeated interventions that might become necessary during its application;
c) the effects of the preliminary medical treatment necessary for carrying out the intervention;
d) the effects and eventual risks the intervention can have upon the patient or the child to be born;
e) the results that can be expected from the application of the procedure;
f) the costs of the applicable procedures;
g) the legal regulations referring to the application of the procedure.

Gamete donation[8]

Gamete donation can be carried out for MAP procedures and for medical research purposes. Donated gametes can exclusively be used for the purpose for which they were donated. No compensation can be requested or provided for the donation of gametes. The necessary and certified costs and loss of income of the donor that occurred connected to the donation should be refunded according to the conditions and the extent defined in the decree of the Minister of Welfare.

Gametes can be donated for the purposes of MAP procedures by competent persons who have not yet turned 35, and who conform to the conditions defined in a separate Act.

Legal status of the *in vivo* and in vitro embryo

Article 54 of the Hungarian Constitution provides that everyone has an intrinsic right to life and human dignity, of which no one can be arbitrarily deprived. By mentioning life and dignity in parallel and in one phrase, the Hungarian Constitution is peculiar in providing the ground for interpreting life and dignity as two aspects of the constitutional concept of individuality - physical and spiritual.

Reference to the concept of human dignity plays an important role in the Hungarian abortion debate, much as reference to privacy and liberty does in the American legal debate on abortion. Nevertheless, it is not clear what is the content of "human dignity" in Hungarian constitutional theory. The meaning of human dignity is not necessarily identical with the concept of the right to self-determination. Dignity can be interpreted as the maxim of being treated as an "end" rather than a "means", or being respected by others. Moreover, based on the constitutional theory that emphasizes the duty of the state to protect "objective rights", dignity is partially independent of the individual's own perceptions of his/her dignity.

Since the political and economic transition, the Hungarian Constitutional Court has twice provided an opinion on the status of the human embryo in respect to abortion. Firstly in 1991 and for the second time in 1998. In the second opinion of the Court[9] while emphasizing the duty of the state with respect to the fetus' right to life, the court also realized that there is a constitutional right, based on the right to dignity, which is broad enough to encompass the pregnant woman's right to self-determination. Balancing these two requirements is the crux of the problem. The Court emphasized that neither an entire ban on abortion, nor the unrestricted self-determination of women would conform to the constitution. Furthermore, the Court recognized that the Hungarian law is not the only one in which, apart from medical necessity and moral, legal indications (e.g. rape), there is a general ground for abortion that is based on the grievous general crisis or mental crisis of the woman. Since there are no established standards to assess such conditions, it is usually the pregnant woman who declares the presence of such a crisis. The Court noted that any determination of distress not based on her assessment would constitute a massive intrusion into the woman's privacy.

The Court emphasized that "grievous crisis" needs to be analyzed in a broader context. In 1992 the Hungarian law[10] adopted a definition of "grievous crisis" that is stricter than the mere statement by the woman of her own assessment of her condition. In this respect, the Hungarian law is stricter than, for instance, the French law. Furthermore, by including the issue of the fetus's endangerment as also a matter of "grievous crisis" the Hungarian law leaves open two options. First is that the woman's and the fetus' crises have to produce a conjunctive condition; second that the woman's crisis alone could be used as a basis for allowing abortion. The latter was, in fact, accepted for use.

In 1998 the Court noted the European tendency to shift from the "objective indications" model, where the indications of a grievous crisis can be monitored by an outsider, to a "subjective indications" model, in which the pregnant woman's statement of her crisis constitutes the basis of permission to abort. Nevertheless it noted that a request to the pregnant woman to disclose the reasons behind her crisis is not a disproportionate restriction of her right to self-determination, if the state-protected right of the fetus hangs in the balance. Here there seems to be a hidden message. The Court realized that radical restriction on the scope of "grievous crisis" would not fit into the current European tendencies in legal theory and interpretation. Nevertheless, the Court wanted to give a gesture of support to the pro-life petitioners.

The Hungarian Constitutional Court often gained inspiration from the decisions of the German Constitutional Court. When analyzing the justification and the scope of the grievous crisis situation the Hungarian Court compared the fundamental inferences between the "undue burden test" as it has been interpreted in the American Casey case and in the second German Abortion Case.

> (The) unreasonable burden standard is justified because in the light of the unique relationship between mother and child, prohibiting abortion does not end with

the imposition of a duty to refrain from violating the right of another.

In the second abortion case the Hungarian Court sharply opposed the American judicial interpretation of the "undue burden test" that requires the State to prove that the legislative restriction on abortion does not amount to undue burden imposed on women. Instead of this line of reasoning the Hungarian Court focused on the justification of the grievous crisis situation by stating that the burden of proof rests not on the state but on the pregnant woman and she has to prove her qualified interest that amounts to a form of undue burden in order to request legitimate abortion. .

Research on the human embryo[11]

Research on the human embryo is considered as a sensitive question and prohibited in many European countries (e.g. Germany, France). In the Hungarian Health Act (Act No. CLIV 1997. Chapter VIII.), however, embryo research is permitted under certain circumstances:

1. The research should be based on the Hungarian Reproduction Committee's permission.
2. The research proposal can be approved only at a health care provider or a research institute having the appropriate professional conditions.
3. An embryo can be used only for those research purposes which specified in the Health Act.
4. Embryos cannot be created for research purposes, only embryos created in MAP procedures can be used for research and experiments, either on the basis of the decision of those entitled to decide, or in the case of damage of the embryo.
5. An embryo cannot be implanted in the body of an animal, human and animal gametes cannot be fertilized with each other.
6. The embryo on which experiments were carried out cannot be implanted into the human body, and cannot be kept alive for more than 14 days - the period of freezing and storage is not included in the duration of the experiment and the period following that.
7. Procedures directed to the choice of the sex of the descendant before birth can only be applied in case of recognition of sex dependent hereditary illness, respectively for the prevention of development of such illness.

Further protection of the embryo is prescribed under article 185 of the Health Care Act when, in the case of multiple pregnancy, the number of embryos can be reduced only if there is a strong and specified medical indication.

Surrogate motherhood

Pregnancy and child delivery is so profoundly attached to the concept of motherhood, that surrogacy is regarded as the most resisted agreement in the field of assisted procreation. While a male's mere financial and social contribution as a husband requires no justification in the legislation, neither does the wife's 'mere child delivery' of the embryo conceived in vitro with her husband's sperm and an egg donor's egg but, when the social mother is "just" a genetic mother but not gestational mother, laws usually formulate harsh prohibitions. In the time of such profound changes in procreation it is interesting that it seems evident to most legislators that gestational motherhood is the "real" form of motherhood. If a woman delivers a child created with her husband's sperm and with a donor's egg no one regards her as a surrogate mother who provides only "shelter" for her husband's baby.

In general, surrogacy is defined as an agreement in which a woman carries a child to term from the initiation of the pregnancy for another woman who becomes a social mother. Fertilization may take place through normal coitus or it may be a consequence of artificial insemination, in vitro fertilization or embryo transfer.

During the 1997 Parliamentary debate one of the most controversial issues was to formulate a position on surrogate motherhood. Surrogacy was a living practice in Hungary even before 1997, in the lack of any explicit legal prohibition. Nevertheless some formal requests for permission were launched, asking the National Science and Research Ethics Council (TUKEB) to allow surrogate motherhood based on the particular aspects of the case. Although some cases were discussed in front of the Council, and even authorized, the overall application of the surrogacy was still difficult to estimate. When the 1997 Health Act included a provision on surrogacy it was often misunderstood that the Act meant to restrict the existing practices but not to permit them. The 1997 Act outlawed commercial surrogacy but allowed altruistic surrogate agreements between relatives. Still there were some practical rather than ethical considerations with respect to the application of this law that resulted in the suspension of the application and to provide two years for working on solutions for the potential family law problems.

The recently introduced dual terminology in the Hungarian language reflects well the distinction between commercial and non commercial form of surrogacy. While commercial surrogacy was named as "béranyaság" (motherhood for salary) the non-commercial surrogacy was named as dajkaterhesseg (that is nurse-mother). This latter expression has no pejorative connotation. On the contrary it creates a pleasant association with the term wet-nursing.

In 1997 the aim of the legislation was to restrict surrogacy to exceptional practice among family members, or where surrogacy is based purely on altruistic motivation. The Act intended to forbid commercial surrogacy. In order to avoid the potential legal conflicts between the couple and the surrogate mother who may change her mind during and after the delivery, the law requires that the surrogate mother has already experienced a pregnancy. The fact that she is a family member would enable her to keep in contact with the child; this could answer the charge that surrogacy is merely womb renting.

By adding protective and defensive elements in the legislation, however the Hungarian law (if it will ever be a law) fell into another trap, namely drawing lines. Fine for those women who have fertile and capable relatives but what of those who may not have such relatives but might have friends? And what of the intrinsic family pressure put on fertile young women to help their infertile cousins, sisters-in-law or nieces?

In the November of 1999 the tension around surrogacy reached a heated pitch when the new Bill became known to the media. It was obvious that the Government elected in 1998 was not sympathetic to the idea of non-commercial surrogacy. No intentions to work on the existing adoption laws were shown, instead the Government chose to outlaw surrogacy in a indirect way, by affirming that only those reproductive services are allowed that are specified in the law. Nevertheless further problems might come since from mere medico-technical point of view surrogacy is nothing but an in vitro fertilization and embryo transfer. In the recent Parliament Act a new paragraph was added as a laconic amendment of the 1997 Health Act by canceling surrogacy from the text of the Parliamentary Act. The Act No CXIX of 1999. came into force in January, 2000. Although opinion survey conducted by the media showed very strong public support for surrogacy, nevertheless the non-commercial surrogacy law was cancelled. Most probably the reasons for the short but influential legislative change was the failure to adopt necessary changes in the family law that would be compatible with surrogacy agreements. An interesting element of this change was that it outlawed all forms of surrogacy but did not ban embryo donation and egg donation.

Conclusion

To the great surprise of those offering a reward to the first Hungarian baby of the year of 2000, the first baby was a test tube baby. There are estimations that the demand for reproductive services is still growing, partly due to advantageous insurance coverage and partly due to advanced and accessible medical technology. In the future further services might be introduced but due the 1999 legislative amendment all of the changes in the technology should be based on legislative affirmation. Recently an *ad-hoc* working group was established with the purpose to design a law on genetic testing and screening even to include some provisions on pre-implantation genetic testing.[12] This form of testing is not yet exercised, though it is already planned in some clinics in Hungary.

Based on the interviews that I conducted with prominent figures involved in vitro fertilization, it is estimated that approximately 4000-5000 embryo transfers are done annually in Hungary. Two thirds of these interventions are done in a private clinic that succeeded in receiving the same insurance coverage for its services as a public hospital. In comparison with other medical services the insurance coverage of assisted procreation, not including the medication, is generous. Financing assisted procreation based on the mandatory health insurance coverage amounts to up to five cycles of treatment or up to one baby born. The pregnancy rate is estimated between 30-40%. The reason for uncertainties is related to the fact that pregnant women after visiting reproductive units or clinics will go for child delivery to different hospitals or obstetrical units and therefore data on the take home baby rate is not always obtained.

The Hungarian reproductive regulations which took into the consideration the lessons drawn from the 1990 British Act, the 1994 French Act and American jurisprudence could be regarded as a good attempt towards transparency. However, it may remain just an isolated attempt if further monitoring and necessary assessment of the success is not established soon. One of the major problems now is the consistent implementation of the Parliamentary Act and the Governmental decree on assisted procreation. The National Obstetrical and Gynecological Institute should urge the commencement of the National Reproduction Registry, which should be later run by the Human Reproduction Committee. Due to the lack of adequate staff and financial resources, however, the Registry still has not started to operate, though it is crucial in order to start monitoring and to establish ethical and legal control over these services. It is fairly unusual that the implementation of the law is so much delayed.

As we should care for the health of the first test tube baby born together with our democracy, transparency of the ethically sensitive procedures, such as various forms of assisted procreation should be guarded, as well.

Notes

1   After the Parliamentary Act No CXIX. of 1999 on "amendment of Acts concerning state administration and land registry, health care and fishing" that modified the 1997 Health Care Act, surrogacy is not any longer mentioned among the reproductive services.

2   The private "Kaáli" clinic that has a clinic in Budapest has also some district clinics in the countryside.

3   T.S. Pongrátz and E. Molnár, Kisgyermekes apák és anyák szülési és családi attitudjei négy európai országban, KSH NKI Kutatási jelentések (Report of the Central Office of Statistics), 1994, 52.sz. 37.

4   M. Donalska and D. Evans, (1996) 'Patients' Perceptions of Assisted Conception Services' in D. Evans (ed) *Creating the Child,* Kluwer Law International, The Hague, pp.291-301.

5   During the Fall of 1996 the Mellon fellowship provided me a unique opportunity to familiarize myself with the French biomedical law. During the Fall of 1996 I studied the normative framework of reproduction in France during the period of 1994-1996.

6   Article 186 of the Health Care Act established the Human Reproduction Commission as a decision making, and controlling body of the Minister for Health.

7   10/1997(V.23.) NM r.) on the Health Care and Science Council (Egészségügyi Tudományos Tanács).

8   Articles 170-174 deal with detailed rules of gamete donation. Here the language of the law is very close to the terminology of the property law.

9   The decision, No 48/1998 (XI.23.) AB decision was published in the Hungarian Official Legal Gazette, No 105/1998 6654-6673.

10   Parliamentary Act No. LXXIX. Of 1992. on the protection of the fetus' life.

11   Detailed provisions are in Article 180.-182 of the Health Care Act.

12   Genetics aspects of the in vitro fertilization had been discussed and published in the collection of interviews of some prominent figures of science and ethics in: Ferenczi Andrea, ed, "Genetika-Génetika" Harmat, Budapest, 1999.

15 Health Council Report on Embryo Research: Perspectives on New Legislation in the Netherlands

WYBO J. DONDORP

Introduction

In view of the situation in the Netherlands, this book is just a bit too early. As it goes into print, the long awaited Bill on the Handling of Human Gametes and Embryos has been sent for review to the State Council. Parliament expects to receive it before the summer of 2000.

The main focus of this contribution will be on a recent advisory report by the Dutch Health Council, which played an important role in the preparatory process leading to the announced bill (Health Council, 1998). According to the most controversial recommendation in this report, new legislation should, under conditions, allow the creation of human embryos for research purposes. This would also affect ratification of the Convention on Human Rights and Biomedicine of the Council of Europe, to which the Netherlands is one of the co-signatories.

The Health Council of the Netherlands

The Health Council of the Netherlands (Gezondheidsraad) is a statutory independent advisory body to the Dutch government. Its task is to provide scientific information on public-health matters relevant to government policy and decision-making. Its assessments include ethical and legal aspects whenever these apply. Members are appointed by the Crown and chosen on the sole basis of their expertise in a field relevant to the work of the Health Council. The Council never convenes in full; the reports are drawn up by ad-hoc committees specifically set up to address a particular question, mostly in response to a request by the government.

The IVF-committee was set up in 1994 in order to provide the then Secretary of State with information relevant to the necessary revision of regulations governing IVF-centres. These regulations stemmed from the mid-eighties, the period in which IVF was introduced in the Netherlands. They had to be updated in order to bring them in line with new developments. The committee was given a broad composition, uniting experts in the fields of obstetrics & gynaecology, reproductive medicine, embryology, epidemiology, medical decision theory, medical ethics and health law. It issued three reports: on ICSI (1996), on regular IVF (1997), and on IVF-related research (1998). The latter report contains an extensive chapter on research using human embryos.

The report on "IVF-related research"

It was not part of the original plan to devote much space and argument to embryo-research, nor did the State Secretary explicitly ask for it. But the two remaining issues for the concluding report, preimplantation genetic diagnosis (PGD) and 'the future of IVF', inevitably led the committee to consider the question whether, in the context of IVF-related research, human embryos might be used as research material, or even be created for that purpose. Given this context, the report deals only with non-therapeutic or 'consuming' embryo-research: pre-clinical research using embryos that are not intended for transfer. According to the committee, therapeutic embryo-research would only be acceptable if the risks for the resulting child can reasonably be overseen. A future example of such therapeutic embryo research might be gene therapy on the embryo.

Ethical and legal perspectives

The report gives an extensive overview of the diverse positions in the debate on the acceptability of consuming embryo research. From an ethical point of view, human embryos are either seen as having the full moral status that persons have, relative or increasing moral status, or no moral status at all (in which case they may still be seen as bearing symbolic value). Among Dutch health lawyers there is broad support for what has been called the theory of progressive legal protection, corresponding with the second of the ethical views just mentioned (Te Braake, 1989; Leenen, 1994).

According to this theory it can be deduced from current law that an increasing level of legal protection is due to the embryo or foetus, corresponding with its developmental stage. In the context of Dutch health law, the theory has its main point of reference in the Termination of Pregnancy Act. By leaving room, under conditions, for legal abortion up to viability but forbidding it beyond that point, the abortion law designates a moment of transition, after which the foetus enjoys a higher degree of legal protection, namely: viability. Another such moment can be inferred from the fact that the Act does not apply to the use of intra-uterine devices in order to prevent pregnancy. This means that implanted embryos are given more protection than non-implanted ones. The former are in the *status nascendi*, whereas the latter are only in the *status potentialis*.

According to the theory, embryos *in vitro* enjoy the same basic level of protection that applies to non-implanted embryos *in vivo*, deriving from the fact that they may develop into a human person. In accordance with this view the developmental limit is set at 14 days, the point at which embryos *in vivo* would be implanted and thus have moved from the *status potentialis* to the *status nascendi*.

Dissenting voices say that the theory does not succeed in deducing from current law that already before implantation embryos deserve legal protection (Sutorius, 1993; Van den Burg, 1994). According these authors, there may be moral reasons for protecting preimplantation embryos, but the argument for doing so cannot be derived from the existing legal framework. This is seen as a reason for pushing ahead with legislation defining the legal status of the human embryo. There is broad consensus about the need for such legislation, but efforts in this direction have until now remained without tangible result.

History of legislation

In the mid-eighties the Health Council was asked to advise the government on the then new technology of IVF and its implications. In a series of reports, the Council took the view that research with spare embryos should be possible in exceptional cases, requiring a major health issue to be at stake. No room should be made for specially creating embryos for research purposes, as that, according to one of these reports, would amount to a 100% instrumentalization of human embryos. The National Ethical Review Board (KEMO) took a different position a few years later. In the context of reviewing a protocol on PGD this committee argued that proper pre-clinical research in the fields of PGD and ART might require the use of specially created embryos, and that this should perhaps not be ruled out without at least seriously looking at the consequences.

After much parliamentary discussion, the coalition government of socialists and Christian Democrats presented a very restrictive bill on embryo research in 1992. It prohibited virtually all embryo research, with the main exception of therapeutic research, defined as promoting the healthy development of the embryo in question. The exception was meant to make room for PGD. It is a fine example of the hypocrisy of wanting to make use of results obtained in other countries of research one would not allow in one's own.

In 1995 a new coalition without the Christian Democrats withdrew the restrictive embryo bill of its predecessor. In a memorandum, parliament was given an outline of what the government had in mind as a replacement for it. A new bill was announced, based upon the theory of progressive legal protection and very much in line with the earlier recommendations of the Health Council. It would allow consuming embryo research under strict conditions:

- surplus embryos only,
- no other means for obtaining the results,
- 14-day limit,
- a major health issue must be at stake.

The memorandum specifies this last condition by saying that the research must be in the fields of (in)fertility, ART, or congenital or hereditary diseases (thus restricting the possible health issues major enough to outweigh objections against using human embryos).

Finally, the memorandum contains a general remark on the government's intention to prohibit such applications of embryo research as cloning, the creation of hybrids and chimaeras, and manipulation of the germ line.

Standpoint of the committee

Against the background of these earlier discussions, what is the position taken in the Health Council's recent report on IVF-related research? The committee (which was entirely different from the one reporting in the eighties; nor was it in any way committed to upholding the conclusions of those earlier reports) starts out by saying that the debate on moral status cannot be decided by independent arguments. Each of the views that can be taken ultimately depends on a particular world-view, religious or non-religious, which cannot as such be vindicated. However, an argument against the 'full status view' is that this position, though not less respectable in itself, is inconsistent with the ethical and legal scope given in our society for abortion, the use of intra-uterine devices as contraceptives, and with acceptance of surplus embryos in IVF-practice.

The committee's own view is as follows. The embryo, as a beginning form of human life, has a certain value by virtue of which it deserves to be treated with respect. On the other hand, this value is not absolute, and may be overridden if other, morally more imperative, interests are at stake. This is to say that embryo research can be acceptable, but also that it always requires justification. It must be clear that the research is absolutely necessary in order to obtain results that may be expected to be of great importance for human health. A further implication is that no more embryos are to be used than are strictly necessary for the research.

Noting the growing international consensus in favour of the 14-day limit, the committee observes that the basis of this consensus is pragmatic rather than argumentative. However, given the fact that human embryos cannot, until now, be cultured for more than a week, it sees no reason to pronounce upon this.

Only surplus embryos?

An important point of discussion was whether the committee should stick to the earlier Health Council view that no embryos should be created for research purposes.

The report acknowledges that there is a moral difference between designating surplus embryos for research and creating them especially for that purpose. But what makes for this difference is not the nature of the use. Using surplus embryos is no less instrumentalizing than is using embryos that are specially created as research material. Nor is it the case that 'being surplus' would affect the status of the embryo in a way that would not count for embryos produced as part of the research. Being surplus does not mean that the embryo deserves less respect or protection. If there is a difference, it must lie in the intention with which embryos of either kind are being produced. Surplus embryos are produced with the intention of allowing the embryo to develop into a child. As this is no longer a realistic possibility (otherwise, the embryo would not be surplus), the choice is between either allowing it directly to perish or else to use it in research. In the other case, the embryo is produced exclusively as research material.

An interesting discussion is one of the meetings, which has not made it into the report, was whether it is correct to say that in the context of IVF embryos are created with the intention of allowing them to develop into a child. Since it is accepted from the outset that some embryos will never be transferred, this is at least not the intention with which every single embryo is produced. Would it not be more accurate to say that, instrumental to the establishment of pregnancy, a number of embryos are being created large enough to ensure optimal results by subsequently selecting some of them for transfer? If this were correct (as I think it is), those opposing special production would have a hard time explaining why they do accept current IVF practice. Some, of course, do not, which is at least consistent.

Without pursuing this line, the committee argued that the value of human embryos should be a *prima facie* reason for not creating them as research material. However, since the value of the embryo is relative, this reason can be overridden. Just as embryo research in general, special production of human embryos for research purposes may be acceptable, but requires justification.

Conditions for the creation of embryos for research purposes

According to the report, creation of human embryos for research purposes can only be justified if the research is expected to yield essential information relevant to a major health issue, which cannot be obtained otherwise.

An example would be the pre-clinical evaluation of the efficacy and safety of *in vitro* maturation and cryopreservation of human oocytes. There is a major health issue involved in the further development of these techniques (improving IVF, reducing risks and burdens related to the procedure). Furthermore, pre-clinical evaluation of the relevant techniques is prerequisite for their introduction in clinical research. Thirdly, the information the research is expected to yield cannot be obtained by other means (animal models, use of surplus embryos).

A final, but essential, condition for research using specially created embryos is that the gametes, especially the oocytes, are obtained in a morally acceptable way.

Interests of oocyte donors

Is it morally acceptable to ask healthy women to subject themselves to the burdens and risks of IVF-treatment in order to donate some of their oocytes, not for treating others, at least not directly, but for research? On this point the committee was divided. Some members thought that this should at least not be ruled out in principle. They drew on the analogy with recruiting healthy subjects for other types of scientific research involving a certain health risk. Others found it completely unacceptable even to make this request. Anyhow, it is unlikely that many women would be willing to undergo hormone stimulation in order to donate oocytes for research. The committee sees three alternative routes: asking IVF-patients, using non-fertilized oocytes and asking women undergoing gynaecological operation permission for harvesting any mature oocytes. Each of these routes may yield some oocytes, but none of them is without problems.

Research for which immature oocytes could be used (as in research on *in vitro* maturation) can be expected to meet with less difficulty in obtaining those cells in a sufficient number. Nor would any member of the committee object to asking women to donate some of their immature oocytes.

Recommendations

The committee recommends that all embryo research protocols should be reviewed centrally. The Central Committee doing this review should use the following criteria:

- a major health issue must be at stake for which the research can be expected to yield essential information
- the research must be scientifically sound
- there must be no other means for obtaining the information
- no more embryos should be used than strictly necessary
- no embryos should be created if surplus embryos can be used
- there should be proper procedures of information and consent
- embryos used for research may not be transferred.

According to the report, the announced legislation should not contain a ban on the creation of embryos for research. It warns that such a ban would stand in the way of a responsible introduction of new techniques in ART. If society wants these techniques, in order to be able to offer better and safer assistance in reproduction, it should face the fact that their introduction requires proper pre-clinical research, which may for some procedures involve the use of specially created embryos.

A limited list of acceptable fields of embryo research?

Another Health Council recommendation relevant to the announced legislation was given in the 1997 report on 'Research using human embryonic stem cells'. This report did not answer a request, but was drawn up at the initiative of the President of the Health Council. The report observes that the most promising potential use of human embryonic stem cells (that is: in transplantation medicine) would fall outside the limitative list of acceptable fields of embryo research in the 1995 government memorandum: (in)fertility, ART, and congenital or hereditary diseases. The Health Council recommends not to incorporate any such list in the embryo law, but to stipulate only that a major health issue must be served by the research. Whether a particular protocol would satisfy this condition could be left to the discretion of the Central Committee for research involving Human Subjects (CCMO).

Round of public consultation

In order to find out to what extent these Health Council recommendations are supported in Dutch society, the Ministry of Health initiated a limited round of public consultation (autumn of 1998). The invited organisations (scientific and professional, patient organisations, feminist and religious groups) were asked to state their position on whether or not special production should be legally forbidden and on whether the law should contain a limitative list of acceptable fields of research, as proposed in the government memorandum.

The Health Council's recommendations were fully supported by most of the scientific and professional organisations that were invited. Other groups, however, were more critical. The ART-patients' organisation would only allow infertility research using surplus embryos. Representatives of the churches and other religious groups strongly opposed the idea of allowing the creation of human embryos for scientific purposes. 'Pro life' and feminist groups took a critical position of ART as such and argued for public debate on limiting its use.

Outlook

This book being just a bit too early, I can only conclude my contribution with some tentative remarks about the announced new Bill on the Handling of Human Gametes and Embryos. On the basis of the 1995 memorandum, the new bill can be expected to be much less restrictive than the one presented by the former coalition. It will be constructed around the notion, laid down in the memorandum, that the human embryo is worthy of respect and protection, but that its value is not absolute and can be overridden if a major health issue is at stake. In the memorandum, the scope thus provided for consuming embryo research is limited to 14 days of embryonic development. Given international convergence on this point, there is no reason to expect a different *terminus ad quem* in the announced bill.

It is further clear that all protocols will require a positive verdict of the recently instituted Central Committee for Research involving Human Subjects (CCMO). It remains to be seen whether the bill will limitatively define the fields of investigation for which human embryos may be used, as proposed in the memorandum, or follow the Health Council's recommendation to leave it completely to the Central Committee to decide whether a sufficiently important health issue is served by the research.

With regard to the prohibition on cloning, loosely framed in the memorandum, the bill can be expected to be more precise, following the interpretative statement made by the Netherlands on signing the relevant protocol to the Convention on Human Rights and Biomedicine of the Council of Europe. Whereas article 1 of the protocol prohibits the creation of genetically identical human beings, the statement interprets the notion of a 'human being' as exclusively referring to a human individual as from the moment of birth. This would, under conditions, give scope for non-reproductive cloning for scientific and therapeutic purposes.

Finally, it is difficult to predict how the issue of creating embryos for research will be handled in the bill. The mixed outcome of the round of consultation held to assess public support for the Health Council's report, as well as the fact that most European countries having laws on embryo research tend to be much more restrictive, may be seen by the government as reasons for holding on to its original intention to allow only research with surplus-embryos. That would also clear the way for ratifying the European Convention on Human Rights and Biomedicine, of which article 18 prohibits the creation of embryos for research purposes. The Netherlands is not only one of the co-signatories to this treaty; it has also put much effort in its preparation and would not want unduly to delay ratification.

While, from a political point of view, holding on to the ban proposed in the memorandum might be the most attractive option, ratification of the convention would make it very difficult in the future ever to reconsider the prohibition. With the convention in force, revision would not be a matter of 'simply' changing the law. To the extent that the arguments against the prohibition, as presented by the Health Council and supported by the scientific community, are seen as materially convincing, the government may want to retain room for manoeuvring by making ratification of the convention subject to a proviso on this point. However, such a proviso can only be made if existing legislation provides a point of reference for the diverging position, thus ruling out an unqualified prohibition of creating embryos for research in the announced embryo bill.

We will soon know how the Dutch government has decided. The new bill, though an important milestone, will then, of course, be subject to further parliamentary discussion. Should it, eventually, come to a legal prohibition of creating embryos for research, this may have important consequences for the future development of ART in the Netherlands. It can only be hoped that those who decide will do so after seriously considering, not only the status of the embryo, but those consequences as well.

In its report on IVF-related research, the Health Council has warned for the temptation of looking for easy ways out of this dilemma. One would be: direct testing in clinical experiments of techniques and procedures about the safety of which the prohibited research could provide important information. The Council regards this as unacceptable: "under no circumstances whatsoever may women and children be turned into trial subjects for the sake of protecting embryos". Another easy way out is very familiar but therefore no less objectionable: awaiting results obtained in countries with a more liberal legislation, so as to be able to take the moral high ground while letting others do the "dirty" work. The Council remarks: "prohibiting research on moral grounds while setting one's sights on results of that research to be obtained abroad undermines the credibility of the arguments supporting that prohibition".

References

Braake te, Th.A.M. (1989), 'Experimenten met embryo's. Een gezondheidsrechtelijke benadering', *Tijdschrift voor Gezondheidsrecht*, vol 13, pp. 86-94.
Burg van der, W. (1994), 'De juridische "status" van het embryo: een op drift geraakte fictie'. *Tijdschrift voor Gezondheidsrecht*, vol 18, pp. 386-409.
Health Council of the Netherlands. Committee on *in vitro* fertilization (1998), *IVF-related research*. Rijswijk 1998, publication nr 1998/08E.
Leenen, H.J.J. (1994), *Handboek Gezondheidsrecht. Deel 1: rechten van mensen in de gezondheidszorg*, Alphen aan den Rijn: Samson/Tjeenk Willink.
Sutorius, E.Ph.R. (1993). 'Manipuleren met leven. Preadvies Nederlandse Juristen Vereniging', *Handelingen Nederlandse Juristen Vereniging*, vol 123 part I, pp. 129-329.

16 Legal Approaches in Germany

INGA HANSCHEL

Legislation

The Embryo Protection Act

The regulation of reproductive medicine has been the subject of lengthy and controversial discussions in Germany since as early as the mid-1980's. Following thorough groundwork in numerous workgroups and commissions, the Embryo Protection Act (Embryonenschutzgesetz, ESchG) finally saw the light in 1991, a belated birth as it were. It can be indirectly traced back to the concluding report of the workgroup "In vitro fertilisation, genome analysis and gene therapy" (the so-called Benda Commission) appointed by the Federal Ministry of Justice and the Minister of Research and Technology, as well as papers by the Enquête Commission "Opportunities and Risks of Gene Therapy", set up by the German Parliament. In the end, however, the ESchG did not come to being as an expression of broad unanimity, but as a compromise solution for incompatible, greatly diverging positions. The law's enactment only partially fulfilled the long-standing need for regulation. As an amendment to the Penal Code, the ESchG almost exclusively contains fine-related regulations; a structured regulation of permitted actions, however, was omitted.

When examining this fragmentary corpus of laws, one must take into consideration, however, that the legislative organs were then very much absorbed in regulating the problems at hand in connection with German Reunification.

The necessity for an extensive system of differentiated legal instruments was indeed stressed in the early consultations for the draft bill. A change in the German Constitution (Grundgesetz) would have been required here, however, as to a great extent, regulation in the field of Health Law in reference to medical training and issues concerning the scope of medical remedy was then reserved for the federal states. In the

163

field of Health Law, where state legislation principally has voice, federal legislative competence solely covered measures against public-threatening and contagious diseases in humans and animals, licensing of medical and other health professions and the health industry, the pharmaceutical, remedial, anaesthetic and toxicological industry, as well as the economic security of hospitals and the regulation of nursing fees (article 74, Nr. 19 and 19a of the Constitution). Regulation on the state level, however, could not ensure the desired federal uniformity. In October of 1994, the Constitution was then amended, in as far as "artificial insemination in humans, the studying and artificial altering of hereditary information as well as regulation of the transplantation of organs and tissues" now fell under federal jurisdiction as well. Although the federal legislative body has since then not made use of this possibility, the enactment of an extensive reproductive medical law is being discussed to a greater extent. Serious plans of the present federal government are visible in events such as the colloquium on such a law which the Federal Health Ministry has planned for May 2000 in Berlin.

In formulating the regulations, the legislator had to take the fundamental right to human dignity (article 1 Constitution) and freedom (article 2 Constitution), as well as the right to personality (article 1 in connection with article 2 Constitution) into account, without undermining the fundamental right to freedom of research guaranteed in article 5. In the process, the clear general value decision of the Constitution in favour of human dignity was confirmed, particularly considering the methods of artificial reproduction whose risks – even according to today's knowledge standard – are often difficult to assess.

In vitro fertilisation

Social and medical protection norms in favour of the embryo can be differentiated in the ban in reference to the methods of in vitro fertilisation (IVF).

The former refer to the parental circumstances: it is forbidden to implant a foreign unfertilised egg in a woman, or to remove an embryo before completion of nidation to implant it in another woman. With these regulations, the legislator makes the donation of egg cells and embryos punishable by law.

Persons who carry out artificial insemination on a woman who is prepared to give her child to a third person on a permanent basis after the birth or persons who implant a human embryo in such a woman are also punishable by law. Surrogate motherhood is thus also forbidden, and in turn almost all forms of the female heterologous system. In violation of the named regulations, the women concerned, however, are exempted from punishment.

At most, the transplantation of an egg fertilised in vitro (i.e. according to the ESchG definition of an embryo) to a genetically "foreign" woman would be allowed if, for unforeseen reasons, a transplantation to the woman the egg was removed from is no longer possible. This is neither a case of forbidden donation of an unfertilised egg, nor an embryo donation, as the latter would require the removal of the embryo from the donor. Similarly, it cannot be considered a case of surrogate motherhood, as the woman bearing the child is not prepared to give up the child to a third person.

Unlike the donation of the egg, heterologous sperm donation is permitted, however not the post-mortem donation.

What is more, the ESchG postulates a basic ban on prenatal sex selection. Those "undertaking to artificially fertilise a human egg-cell with a sperm cell which has been selected according to the sex it possesses" are punished by law, the exception here being the selection aimed at preventing serious gender-related hereditary diseases.

From a medical point of view, the legislator seeks to prevent more extreme multiple pregnancies as well as the creation of surplus embryos by prohibiting, for one, the transference of more than three embryos to a woman in the course of one cycle, or the fertilisation of more than three egg cells by means of Gamete Intra Fallopian Transfer. Secondly, the legislator bans the fertilisation of more egg cells than can be transferred to a woman within one cycle.

Research

The ESchG includes extensive prohibition of non-therapeutic research without using the term itself, whereby artificial fertilisation of an egg for any purposes other than the bringing about of pregnancy in the woman who produced the egg, is forbidden. With this regulation, the coming to being of surplus embryos which could be used for research purposes is to be prevented (also see above). Furthermore, the sale, passing on, purchasing or use of an embryo "not serving the purpose of its preservation" are prohibited, as is the effecting of development of an embryo outside of the body for any purpose than that of bringing about a pregnancy.

Punishable by law is also the artificial alteration of the hereditary information of human germline cells, as well as the use of a thus altered cell for fertilisation. This is not valid, however, if it can be excluded that these germline cells will be used for fertilisation. Reservations about this exception are expressed however, that it prevents actual protection as it makes the preliminaries of gene manipulation on humans exempt from punishment. On the other hand, there is a call for relaxation in view of the use of embryonic stem cells.

The development of chimeras and hybrids, as well as cloning (artificially producing the effect that an embryo with the same hereditary information as another embryo, fetus or person, living or deceased, comes to being) is prohibited, whereby the German ESchG does not differentiate between reproductive and non-reproductive cloning. The manipulation of cells following conclusion of cell division (body cells), however, is permitted, as, in this case, the alteration has no effect during cell division and reproduction; somatic gene therapy is thus permissible.

The procedure of cryo-conservation, which according to ESchG as such is not prohibited, continues to be greatly controversial, the objections being that this procedure would lead to a collection of embryos, which could hardly be withdrawn from use as research objects. According to these objections, there remains the danger of great loss by freezing and thawing the embryos, as the embryos would not survive this process. Cryo-conservation is, in any case, relatively insignificant, as the intentional production of surplus embryos is prohibited by the ESchG.

For the procedure of cryo-conservation, artificial fertilisation and embryo transfer, the ESchG provides a medical reservation, as well as a conscience clause which states that no individual is committed to engage in the said procedures. The legal definition of the term "embryo" encompasses the phase as early as the development-capable fertilised egg from the point of cell union and every totipotential cell. Therefore preimplantation genetic diagnosis (PGD) – when practised on totipotential cells – is forbidden, as even the splitting of such a cell to be studied would qualify as the creation of a new embryo with the same hereditary information, thus cloning. In as far as there is the medical possibility of carrying out PGD on non-totipotential embryonic cells as well, this would not be banned as cloning. Controversial, however is the question of whether or not the banning of the misuse of the embryo (by means of use not serving the purpose of its preservation; see above) is an obstacle to such a procedure. Diseases should indeed be discovered by means of PGD; not, however, with the result of therapeutic healing of the embryo, but with the possible consequence of its not being implanted in the uterus, not exactly serving the purpose of its preservation. The use of already sorted cells, taken, for example, from the maternal blood, would change the legal position. In this case, there is no issue of "use" of the embryo, rendering a procedure such as this permissible.

Professional self-regulation

Even before the enactment of the ESchG, the Federal Medical Council was extensively occupied with the issue of assisted reproduction and research on human embryos and filled the existing regulation gap by means of the enactment of professional guidelines. Legislatively allocated leeway must be kept, however, with regulations concerning professional self-regulation. As special legal regulation did not exist, the medical professionals hoped to get around the enactment of a conclusive law with the provision of detailed regulations. In the end, the various regulations did indeed have to be aligned with the federal legislative provisions following enactment of the ESchG. In 1997 in the draft "Professional Guidelines for German Physicians" and related "Guidelines for IVF and Embryo Implantation as a Method of Treating Human Sterility" (henceforth: "Guidelines"), the Federal Medical Council adapted the legal provisions of the ESchG, though modified. These regulations passed as "models" are only valid in the versions released by the individual State medical councils. These do not differ greatly from those provisions on the federal level.

The model professional guidelines provide an extensive ban corresponding to that in the ESchG on research on embryos as well as the creation of human embryos for this purpose. Moreover, it expressly prohibits – here more restrictive than the ESchG – generally the undertaking of diagnostic measures on the embryo prior to implantation in the uterus, i. e. above all, the carrying-out of PGD. The exception to this rule is, however, use for the exclusion of serious gender-specific hereditary diseases. In February of 2000 the Federal Medical Council released a discussion draft for a guideline on PGD, according to which gene analysis could be taken into consideration if there has been as case of a severe hereditary disease in the family involved. PGD should, however, continue to be forbidden following in vitro fertilisation carried for grounds of infertility. According to the Guideline draft, the test would have to be licensed by two Commissions and be restricted to particularly qualified institutions. Exact registration would be obligatory. This exception can as well be found in the ESchG concerning exceptionally permissible sex-selection.

In addition to the provisions of the ESchG, the model professional guidelines only permit the undertaking of artificial insemination for the treatment of sterility and only in accordance with the guidelines.

These differentiate between restricted and unrestricted indications. What is more, carrying out IVF is principally solely permissible within a homologous system; exceptions can be made after the calling-in of a Medical Council Commission, specially set up for this purpose. The most important medical requirement to be fulfilled for exceptionally permissible heterologous sperm donation is that treatment in the homologous system is not possible due to an existing sterility in the male (annex to Guidelines). The doctor's supposed responsibility for the "beneficial development of the child and avoidance of social disadvantages" is cited in the annex as an argument for the regulation. According to this argument, this is principally only possible within the legally acknowledged form of family planning. Illegitimate and legitimate children were treated as equals: however the positive right to extra-marital reproduction was not explicitly expressed.

Unlike the Guidelines, the ESchG solely prohibits the development of the embryo in the body of a woman from whom the egg cell was not taken; the law does not require the persons involved to be married.

Particular legal problems in heterologous systems

The possibility of sperm donation offered in the ESchG leads inevitably to the legal problem of donor anonymity. Does a child who came to being by means of sperm donation have the right to know who his biological father is? In 1989, the Constitutional Court of Germany ruled in a principle decision that the right to personality (article 1, paragraph 1 in connection with article 2, paragraph 1 of the Constitution) encompasses the right to receive knowledge of one's own descent.[1] Based on this fundamental right, a doctor cannot deny a child information concerning the donor if asked to do so. In the light of this, medical confidentiality thought to protect data related to the donor, is considered inferior.

It is thus stipulated in the annex of the Federal Medical Council Guidelines that sperm donation can only be carried out if the donor has expressly given his consent to the child's receiving his name upon request. The biological paternity is crucial for the child's health and that of his own descendants, also the reason for the guideline's prohibiting the use of mixed sperm.

A further controversial problem in connection with heterologous insemination is the civil-legal question of whether or not the child created by means of procedure such as this has a claim to support from the donor. There is a multitude of Supreme Court decisions concerning this issue.[2] The first question is that of the child's legitimacy. A child created by means of heterologous insemination whose mother is married is in principle legitimate. Independent of whether or not he agreed to the creation of the child, the husband thus has the legal obligation to pay child support. The husband's giving of his consent to the creation of a child by means of heterologous insemination is, though, seen as a contractual acceptance of the legal obligation to pay child support for the good of the child. This contractual obligation – as opposed to the legal obligation – does not automatically cease with the establishment of the child's illegitimacy. In the case that the husband himself contests the legitimacy of the child (which is his right), he may draw no further rights and is still obliged to pay child support. If the child, on the other hand, establishes his own illegitimacy, according to the law, the donor would then have to bear the responsibility of child support. This very unsatisfactory result, hardly corresponding to a common understanding of the law, could be avoided by interpreting the husband's consent to the heterologous creation of the child as a contract in favour of the donor, who then has a claim against the husband to be exempted from having to pay child support. Obviously, jurisdiction has yet to deal with this issue in depth. It remains to be seen, if a decision is to be made in this regard in the future.

Health insurance law and costs

The reimbursement for artificial insemination by state health insurance is laid down in the Social Code (Sozialgesetzbuch) V (SGB V), according to which the health insurance pays for "medical measures for the bringing about of a pregnancy" under the condition that this is necessary to bring about a pregnancy, that sufficient prospects of a pregnancy are given and that the persons whose egg and sperm cells are to be used are married and have undergone consultation. Following four failed attempts, sufficient prospects of pregnancy is negated, with the result that the expense of further attempts is not carried by the health insurance.

Solely the treatment of the person insured is taken over by the state and by private insurance companies.

Summary and statement

A closer look reveals that many regulations in the ESchG are less concerned with the protection of the embryo than the protection of "accredited forms of family planning", wording found in the annex of the Federal Medical Council Guidelines, whose principle, however, is also found in the ESchG. This motivation is clearly revealed in the ban on surrogate motherhood.

Negative influence on the emotional development and particular difficulties of the child's self-discovery have by no means been proven in so-called "split motherhood" (different genetic and bearing mothers). Influence of this sort is, however, cited as an argument for the prohibiting of egg and embryo donation. Furthermore, it must be noted that, in view of the fact that sperm donation is permitted, the extensive ban of measures carried out within the female heterologous system contradicts equal rights for men and women guaranteed in the Constitution. The professional guidelines even go so far as to fundamentally prohibit any form of artificially induced pregnancy in non-married couples, the argument being that in an existing partnership, it can be required of the partners fostering the serious wish to have a child, to document this seriousness by means of entering into marriage. According to the Guidelines, carrying out artificial insemination on a single woman, on the other hand, is in principle unjustifiable. Illegitimate children were still today exposed to social disadvantages. No positive right to reproduction resulted from the legal equality of illegitimate and legitimate children. Therefore this equality did not provide legitimisation for doctors to assist non-married couples in receiving artificial insemination - a rather questionable manner of argumentation. Indeed, the right to reproduction resulting from the said equality is to be denied. In adapting the motives of legislation, however, this equality should not be completely disregarded as legislative regulatory orientation. A doctor should thus principally be allowed to carry out artificial insemination on non-married couples according to professional guidelines as well. With rules of conduct such as these, the question arises as well as to what extent a doctor, in his function as such, is obliged to penetrate into the social situation of the partners in regarding the decision about treatment.

Rather remarkable as well in this context is the comment in the annex to the Guidelines which states that a doctor should refrain from carrying out artificial insemination if, after conversations with the partners and their psychological counselling, he reaches the conclusion that existing problems in the relationship cannot be overcome with the birth of a child.

Taking account of the – compared to other European countries – very high research hurdles presented by the ESchG, it would seem desirable to permit at least non-therapeutic research on surplus embryos if their transplantation has been excluded. Even if the creation of embryos solely for research purposes and the intentional creation of surplus embryos as "reserves" for failed transfers - the two cases being difficult to distinguish - continue to be prohibited in the presence of applicable and internationally recognised considerations, surplus embryos could nonetheless come to being through such severe damage that transfer is rendered impossible.

As the destruction of such embryos is inevitable, allowing specified research could be taken into consideration if it served important purposes, several of which could be laid down and/or necessitate consent by an especially established. In certain cases one could come to the conclusion, in considering means and purpose, that the benefit derived from the corresponding research should be given higher priority than protecting from research an embryo which will be destroyed. In these cases, the use of such embryos could be admitted for research purposes. In its report, the "Benda Commission" also expressed its being against such a ban. One must remember, however, that even in lifting such a ban, the number of embryos needed for achieving substantial results would be greatly insufficient.

On the other hand, in discussions on easing the ban on research, one should not disregard that this issue implies possible violation of fundamental values such as human dignity and the right to life. There is always the danger that, given increased opportunities for manipulation of the human gene, the value of human life will be increasingly judged by its genetic characteristics. Thus, each individual case must be subject to particular scrutiny.

The ESchG ban on non-therapeutic research does not extend - as do further bans given in the ESchG and other than the ban on abortion in punishable cases - to acts committed abroad, i.e. doctor and patient can carry out treatment abroad.

The issues tossed up in discussions on research bans demonstrate a clear relation to the problems related to the topic of abortion. Generally permitting PGD could thus help prevent advanced-stage abortions. and the related physical and psychological burden. Indeed, one must not overlook the fact that an at least potential new life comes to being during the splitting of totipotent cells and that the splitting brings a certain risk for the embryo. The latter problem can, however, be taken into account in thorough and informative counselling with the woman involved of the risks of the various procedures. The fact that according to the ESchG, a cloning has taken place with the carrying-out of this method is to be given less weight than the interest in early diagnosis of severe diseases.

Furthermore, there is the issue of whether the restrictive research ban shows a value contradiction to abortion regulations which do not provide the embryo with equally exclusive protection. This view does not consider, however, that it is exactly the particular conflictive situation of the pregnant woman that accounts for the regulations on abortion, to weigh the woman's interest with the embryo's right to life and perhaps to even give it more weight. There is also no inconsistency found in the fact that, in the case of abortion, the embryos can be destroyed (in the case of permitted abortion), whereas the ESchG prohibits *use* not serving the purpose of preservation, as according to general opinion, *destruction* is not prohibited by the ESchG; it is no case of misuse.

To summarise, one can say that the ESchG reflects the general legal-political morale in Germany, which still clearly resists research on human embryos and tends to be characterised by its mistrust in new artificial reproduction technologies.

The enactment of the ESchG, however, by no means ended the debate in Germany on artificial reproductive medicine and research on human embryos. On the contrary; the fragmented character of the legislation leaves several questions open, above all it lacks, for reasons already mentioned, structured regulations of permitted acts. For this reason, studies initiated by the federal government have been carried out since 1995 into the extent to which an extensive law concerning artificial reproduction medicine is actually required. Since then, two commissioned reproductive medical scientists, among others, have been dealing with this issue in two expert reports and a working group made up of members on federal and state levels. Regulation of the legal relationship between child, mother, husband and sperm donor in heterologous sperm donation seems absolutely necessary. Regulation of pre-implantation genetic diagnosis, taking, for instance, the Federal Medical Council's Guideline draft of February of 2000, and treatment of surplus embryos, above all concerning cryo-conservation, is desirable, particularly in view of these explosive issues.

Notes

1   Constitutional Court, decision of 31.1.1989 – 1 BvL 17/87.
2   Constitutional Court, decision of 3.5.1995 Neue Juristische Wochenschrift (NJW) 1995, 2028; decision of 3.5.1995 NJW1995, 2031; decision of 12.7.1995 NJW 1995, 2921.

References

Deutsch, E. (1999), *Medizinrecht*.
Koch, H.-G. (2000), ‚Rechtliche Voraussetzungen und Grenzen der Forschung an Embryonen' (forthcoming), *Geburtshilfe und Frauenheilkunde*.
Laufs, A., Uhlenbruck, W. (1999), *Handbuch des Arztrechts*.
Neidert, R. (1998), ‚Brauchen wir ein Fortpflanzungsmedizingesetz?', *Medizinrecht*, pp. 347-353.

17 Regulating Reproductive Technologies: Ten Years Down the Tube?

DEREK MORGAN

I. Medical law

Medical law is in large part a process of *naming, blaming, claiming and declaiming*. Naming - is this person ill, unwell, chronic, acute etc; blaming – exploring the role of caring for oneself, one's responsibilities for health care, particularly, whether we are responsible for our own health but also the state responsibility for provision of health care and our collective responsibility for other nations' health; claiming - what are our entitlements to health care, of access to services? and declaiming –about saying who we are and whom we want to become, giving a moral and symbolic emphasis to law.[1] This taxonomy is suggested as appropriate for a very specific historical moment; one in which the late C20th has seen an inversion of the mood that Orlando Figes has described as that of the immediate post revolutionary period in Russia. Figes has characterized that as an "age of optimism in the potential of science to change human life and, paradoxically at the same time, an age of profound doubt and uncertainty about the value of human life itself in the wake of the destruction of the first world war".[2] The late C20th in contrast, (in which a global concern with ethics appears to have become its defining stigmata)[3] has come to view scientific 'progress' with a profound skepticism - at least as to the human and economic costs entailed - while setting in place of this 'profound doubt' as to the value of human life (at least in individualized, Westernized societies, and in respect at least of individual, Westernized lives) a rededication, a reaffirmation, of its individual sanctity or sacredness.[4] It is against this background that this examination of the regulation of reproductive technologies takes place.

Recent authoritative accounts of regulation [5] have had little to say about the emergence of 'new' health technologies and their social and statutory reception. Conceptually, there is nothing that necessarily dictates that access to and control over health technologies could not or should not be subject to the same or a similar analysis.[6] The work so far done has been of a predominately descriptive nature,[7] whether in the UK,[8] Europe,[9] or the common law world.[10] Insofar as these accounts have considered seriously the emergence and expansion of health technologies, they have done so within discrete disciplinary boundaries; little work has sought to locate an account of *regulating* innovative health technologies, such as reproductive medicine and genetics, within changing constitutional frameworks, the responsibilities of holistic government,[11] related to questions of social exclusion,[12] and the emergence of demands for supra-national regulation of bio-medicine and the identification of appropriate fora which have come to occupy the international community in the last decade.[13]

The statutory regulation of assisted conception - that, for example, now adopted in the United Kingdom and said by many commentators to provide a model for other jurisdictions and one which is indeed appealed to by many - is but one of a number of possible models of regulation. In this essay I do not intend exhaustively to review the experience with that statutory model, nor to provide a detailed comparison with the form or substance of other models which have emerged over the past 10 years in other European jurisdictions or internationally.[14] Rather, I want to begin an examination of what it implies to speak of *models of regulation*. I shall suggest a number of background philosophical and specifically sociological questions upon which models of regulation must be predicated, and then with two examples, illustrate some of the questions which this statutory scheme has had to consider in the last decade.

II. The challenges of regulating medical practices

There is a variety of different instruments which can be and are employed to regulate the activities of scientific and technical societies, each of which requires us to examine what is meant by 'regulation'. Thus, one might distinguish at least between;

1   formal (state) law; specially formulated legal principles and norms applied to the subject matter in questions, or to the processes which are the subject matter;

2   formal (state) law which is of general applicability;

3 informal, general or specific law; such as professional codes of practice or discipline which may be either promulgated under a general state law which regulates professions, or professionals of a particular kind, or subject to special and specific qualifications or which may be adopted voluntarily by the professional body concerned and which may be either of a general directive kind or a specific mandatory provisions which covers certain defined activities rather than (say) providing only the conditions of good professional practice;

4 moral suasion;

5 the market.

And in respect of each type of approach, we may ask to whom or to what are 'the rules' of the regulation directed. In each case, again, it is necessary to consider the relationship between;

- the international community
- the nation state
- 'individual' patients or consumers
- scientific and technical practitioners
- resulting 'social practices' with respect to relationships between people.

And, when assessing novel medical technologies – such as assisted conception - and their judicious introduction into therapeutic practice and the applicable form or nature of regulation, it is appropriate to distinguish a number of 'phases'. These include

- the developmental phase;
- the human subjects trial phase;
- the phase considering the incorporation of the technology into health care; and
- the diffusion phase.[15]

As European countries increasingly debate questions arising from in vitro fertilization and embryo research it is apparent that general *agreement* is emerging, both within the scientific community and European institutions that common, core approaches are desirable.[16] Unless there is to be a 'harmonization downwards' (which could be either towards more restrictive or more liberal or radical approaches) it is apparent that if research centers in different countries are to engage in successful, co-operative projects, then some common ethical norms, backed by harmonized sanctions, are essential. Against this background, Albin Eser has suggested that legal initiatives may be required for one or more of four reasons, which correspond roughly to the taxonomy of 'naming, blaming, claiming and declaiming' that I identified earlier.[17] These 'initiatives' he proffers are;

A symbolic function of law; declaring certain values and interests as worth protection against any infringement (of which prohibitions on altering the structure of the nucleus of an embryo and protecting the life of the unborn fetus are commonly given as paradigm examples);

A protective function; providing sanctions for abuses within the bioethical field, and for minimizing risks to patients and significant others affected by the application of biotechnology - such as potential children who might be born following assisted conception;

A regulative or declarative function; there is probably no legal system with a comprehensive biomedical law. The legal status of many bioethical practices is unclear in the absence of parliamentary intervention, which is seen or appealed to as securing clarity and certainty in handling controversial areas of bioethics;

A technical function of law; for stabilizing confidence between physician and patient by providing reliable rules for their relationship. One example of this might be ground rules relating to access to lawful abortion facilities, another dealing with aspects of confidentiality in respect of genetic knowledge obtained during the course of pre-natal or ante-natal screening, and a third in the (non) disclosure of the identity of gamete donors to children born as a result of assisted conception.

In each country of Europe, including Eastern Europe, similar questions arise with respect to law, medicine and bioethics. But there are differences of a philosophical, economic, social, political and even geographical nature which are not easily (even if desirably) bridged. The parallel between explosive political change within and across Europe and the rapid developments in biomedical sciences and their impacts on the fields of law, ethics and human rights give rise to challenges on at least three levels.[18]

Human rights

What is the meaning, for example, of a 'fundamental right to human life', and in what way(s) is this question metamorphosed by biotechnology? What is meant by the European Convention on Human Rights' guarantee (in Article 12) of the right to 'marry and found a family' and how do substantive and procedural barriers to access to biotechnology impinge on that 'right'? Reconciliation of advances in medicine and science with values expressed through human rights is necessary to preserve the bioethical balance; to ensure that the risks to patients, providers and the subjects of biotechnology are minimized. Laws, administrative regulations and professional codes of conduct must be carefully scrutinized to elaborate the effects they set out to achieve, whether they achieve those and only those ends, and whether there are other, unintended, unforeseen or unforeseeable effects.[19]

Democracy and public choice

How should these difficult issues be mediated; towards consensus, a toleration of moral pluralism, or within the dictates of one dominant philosophical approach? What is the fulcrum of the bioethical balance? What institutional structures are used, proposed or necessary to articulate and effect these determinations of public choice?

The rule of law

A fundamental question which arises for any jurisdiction is whether there is any existing law which regulates biomedical practice, research and development and whether it is satisfactory in assisting our responses to ethical dilemmas posed by biotechnology; is it too accommodating or too antagonistic?

Possible responses to these challenges, an understanding of the intellectual forces which have produced them, and the mediation of differences of form and substance comprise what I have elsewhere called *biomedical diplomacy.*[20] This concept can be located within a wider theoretical construct, identifying shifts in the nature of philosophical practices, and the development and deployment of new forms of regulation which both supplement and represent a challenge to the increasing juridification (the danger of the uncritical and unreflective appeal to and of law),[21] and of social and technical practices.

Biomedical diplomacy attempts to identify and negotiate 'tragic choices'[22] which have to be constantly (re)mediated; it examines how modern biomedicine requires the re-negotiation and regulation of existing boundaries of risk, technology and power, and how it attempts to achieve this at the level of individual state. This it does at a time of enormous geo-political, economic, and epistemological upheaval; a global concern with ethics appears to have become the defining stigmata of the late C20th[23] pluralism is replacing old certainties and the generic 'patient' is disappearing.[24] Biomedical diplomacy, negotiating the tragic choices, is in part necessary to ensure that we retain a belief that we shall be privy to what the outcomes of individual choices will be. Law is part of what might be understood to be comparative public policy making and responses to the forces of globalization; we are here concerned to examine the role of law in regulating biotechnology in what Ulrich Beck has called 'the risk society'.[25]

III. Assisted conception and the risk society

Ulrich Beck cautions against the dangers of uncontrolled or unregulated uses and developments of science and technology. He has suggested that while the latest research results constantly open up possible new applications, because this happens at such a rapid, exponential rate, the process of implementation is practically uncontrolled. A variant on this that I would add is that where it is controlled, countervailing arguments are more easily marshaled on the basis of benign experience or supposed individuation of consequences. Accordingly, while medicine supposedly serves health, it has in fact 'created entirely new situations, has changed the relationship of humankind to itself, to disease, illness and death, indeed, it has changed the world'.[26]

One of Beck's interlocutors has recently distilled the concept of 'risk society' in a way that may be more accessible for a legal audience. Anthony Giddens has cautioned that the idea of 'risk society' does not as might be thought, suggest a world which has become more hazardous, Rather, it is a society increasingly preoccupied with the future (and also with safety), which generates the notion of risk; the use of 'risk' is taken to represent a world 'which we are both exploring and seeking to normalize and control'.[27] In this understanding, 'risk society' suggests a society which increasingly 'lives on a high technological frontier which absolutely no one completely understands and which generates a diversity of possible futures'.[28] The origins of the risk society can be traced to two fundamental transformations each connected to the increasing influence of science and technology although not wholly determined by them.   'The first transformation can be called *the end of nature*; and the second *the end of tradition.*'[29]   The 'risk society' is one that creates *manufactured risk*; 'science and technology create as many uncertainties as they dispel - and the uncertainties cannot be 'solved' in any simple way by scientific evidence.'

The unprecedented speed of change in medical practices and the radical uncertainty and anxiety which has been an accompaniment to this, has generated new, (self-producing) uncertainty;

> ... we are living in a state of epistemological turbulence ...   It is as though Durkheim's motto has been reversed.   Rather than studying social phenomena as if they were natural phenomena, scientists now study natural phenomena as if they were social phenomena.[30]

There are those who believe that work in present biotechnical research and associated infertility treatment services is like playing alchemy in the crucible of the genetic future.   They suspect that the atoms will enter new, unforeseeable and dangerous trajectories and take on vectors and forces that cannot now be understood.   In this vision, under the eye of the biotechnological clock we are moving towards some alchemical Armageddon in which the horsemen of the apocalypse become the cavalry charge of the chromosomal chemists.   For some, the sanctioning of research on human pre-embryos signals that the orders for that charge have already been given, and that the slippery slopes of disaster and destruction have already been tested and will exercise an inexorable gravitational pull.[31]

In parallel with this are doubts that have consistently been voiced about the wisdom of investing resources so heavily in the 'reproduction revolution'.[32]   Against a background of serious, if contested, concern about the continuing rapid development and growth of population size in certain quarters of the globe and more explicit, feminist arguments about such technological fixes to the perceived problem of infertility and childlessness,[33] there are fears that present imperatives address at several levels the wrong problem and certainly propose the wrong solutions.

The public policy challenge is to obtain all the benefits and advantages of these developments in reproductive technology but to control these developments and guide them in the directions that we want.   One of the major difficulties will be to identify the unwanted or unwarranted consequences, but a prior problem will be to agree upon which consequences are unwanted or unwarranted and how these are best to be avoided and minimized and what the opportunity costs are of having identified and chosen to regulate in one way rather than another. The types of control which could be envisaged include i) a private ordering approach, based upon individual control, responsibility and power; ii) professional self-regulation and control, through the medical profession, local research and institutional review committees, which has been a hallmark of medical regulation and supervision for many centuries; iii) community control, through national ethics committees and the courts; iv) legislative and regulatory control; v) a combination or blending of one or more of these approaches. Whichever is chosen will reflect the perceived judgment of the proper role of the state in assisted conception, standing here as a surrogate for or a lieutenant to science and technology more generally. As McLean has suggested, 'human reproduction is, in part regulated by law because it is seen as more than a merely private matter'.[34]

IV. The Regulation of assisted conception

Most states have on examination, eventually concluded that some form of regulatory control usually through specially framed and implemented legislation is preferable to no regulation, although the nature of that regulation and review differs markedly. Yet, it is fascinating and remarkable that so few common law countries - in which we might also include the various jurisdictions of the US - have regulatory legislation dealing comprehensively with facets of assisted conception. Of course, it is true that wise government does not always legislate at the first opportunity, and the global nature of the reproduction revolution makes the absence of attention to concerted international legislation perhaps more surprising than would be its presence.[35] The major jurisdictions of Canada, Australia, Japan and the US have no (federal) legislation (where that lies within the federal government's authority) and in the absence of that relatively few individual states have moved to fill that vacuum.

Secondly, it is remarkable - with what seems to be increasing frequency - how often one reads of the HFEA as being viewed as the appropriate regulatory model to have introduced when comparative assessments of models of regulation are assayed. The United Kingdom HFE Act:

> provides the first attempt in English law to provide a comprehensive framework for making medical science democratically accountable. Its

interest therefore arises both from the solutions it adopts for particular issues and from the model of regulation on which it builds…. The nature of the forum in which the debates about infertility treatment and embryo research are to be carried out is structured by a complex web of discretion, restraints, control and accountability.[36]

Statutory regulation might be thought to bring a number of significant advantages and some possible disadvantages, which include those set out in Table 17.1.

Table 17.1 Statutory regulation

Advantages	Disadvantages
Certainty, stability and consensus forming	Moral hazard and slippery slopes; legitimacy
Political advantages; democratic accountability and legitimacy	Definitional questions (e.g.; what is a 'gamete'; cloning) and transitional problems (from self or voluntary regulation to statutory regulation)
Statute with Code allows flexibility to respond to developments *after reflection*	Cost ('a tax on the infertile')
Remove or reduce 'procreative tourism' and 'forum shopping'	Legitimacy; conflicts of interest, 'capture'
Biomedical Diplomacy	Adverse reactions (e.g. of patients) to compulsion (e.g. counseling) and soft paternalism

Some 10 years ago, when the Bill that was to become the 1990 Act was being debated, clinical freedom was then prayed in aid of relieving some aspects of assisted conception, such as GIFT, from the purview of the then to-be-created Human Fertilisation & Embryology Authority. As Lord Mackay of Clashfern, the Lord Chancellor of the day said in debate;[37]

> we think that licensing this technique [GIFT] except where it involves donated gametes when it does clearly fall within the scope of the licensing arrangements, would be to take a first step which could logically lead to a much larger degree of statutory regulation of medical treatment...

I thought that that judgment in that absolute form was wrong at the time and I remain unpersuaded that in this small field, this limited corner of medical practice, that there is not room for greater oversight of further aspects of assisted conception. However, in concluding an overview of the 1990 Act I wrote with Bob Lee that;

> That the Human Fertilisation and Embryology Act is incomplete does not mean that it is unwelcome. But it will not be the last word on the subject.[38]

These words, written in the spring of 1989 have indeed come to bear some fruit just ten years later. And they were written before the name of Diane Blood had ever appeared on our computer screens. In turn, Mrs Blood has left the trail of her name in the corridors of the Human Fertilisation & Embryology Authority and its legal advisors, even before the coming into effect of Article 12 and 8 of the European Convention on Human Rights as envisaged by the Human Rights Act 1998.

Recall that Article 12 provides that 'Men and women of marriageable age have the right to marry and found a family...'; and Article 8 that '(1) Everyone has the right to respect for his private and family life ...', which may be abrogated only in limited circumstances.[39] A recent commentary on the Human Rights Act concluded one of its sections on 'future issues' by suggesting that;

> When Diane Blood sought to use her dead husband's sperm to conceive a child she succeeded on the basis of European Community free movement law. Had the Human Rights Act 1998 been in force she may have succeeded more easily by invoking Articles 12 and 8.[40]

I choose this example for this important reason. Immediately after the Blood case the Government commissioned a review from Professor Sheila McLean of the Consents Provisions of the HFEA.[41] Thereafter, Professor Brazier's committee reviewed the operation of the provisions of that Act and the Surrogacy Arrangements Act 1985.[42] The time may be approaching when it is right for a wider review of the Human Fertilisation and Embryology Act. This is necessary in an innovative field such as this anyway, but also better to be able to understand the nature and type of regulation which is properly called for in this sensitive area. I am strengthened in this belief by the recent conclusions of the review by the Human Genetics Advisory Commission and the HFEA in their consultation report *Cloning Issues in Reproduction, Science and Medicine*.[43] At para 9.7 they observe

> ... because the pace of scientific advances in the area of human genetics, the HGAC and the HFEA believe that the issues need to be kept under regular review to monitor scientific progress. We therefore recommend, that the issues are re-examined again in, say, five years time, in the light of developments and public attitudes towards them in the interim.[44]

Mutatis mutandi assisted conception as whole.

V. Specific issues down the tube

Let me now turn to two specific issues that can be used, and are used here only in an illustrative fashion to disclose some of the trials of working with a statutory scheme of regulation; the two questions are the recovery and storage of ovarian tissue and gametes and the posthumous use of recovered gametes. I am not to be taken to imply, of course, that similar issues or difficulties might not arise under some other form of regulation; rather I use them merely as examples of the continuing tensions between scientific advances and the demands of law.

The legality of taking and storing ovarian tissue and gametes

Writing ten years ago Bob Lee and I had observed that there were some matters, not included in the Act, which would give rise to their own difficulties. For example, we noted that

> The Act nowhere deals with the special position of minors and gamete donation. It is presumably left to the common law, or to guidance which [HFEA] is minded to offer in the Code. There may be good reason to distinguish between the donation of sperm and the donation of eggs, particularly in relation to minors. ... A specific exception could perhaps have been considered in the course of therapeutic surgery, ...

The relevant provisions to consider here are those of the Human Fertilisation & Embryology Act 1990 ss 4(1), 12, 14 and Sch 3 (consents); s 2(2), sch 3 para 8(1) (storage) and the HFEA Code of Practice, paras 3.39 - 3.42.

The general rules in relation to the removal and storage of ovarian tissue and testicular tissue are set out in guidance from the HFEA, given their understanding of the common law and the provisions of the HFEA.

Oocyte Preservation and Ovarian Tissue Storage A person who keeps or uses gametes in contravention of the Act is guilty of offence. If ovarian tissue contains gametes as understood by the HFEA then the licensing provisions of the Act apply and a storage license is generally required. Gametes are understood by the HFEA to be;

> ... a reproductive cell, such as an ovum or a spermatozoon, which has a haploid set of chromosomes and which is able to take part in fertilization with another of the opposite sex to form a zygote.[45]

If the ovarian tissue which is taken does *not* contain gametes as understood by the HFEA (and a practical difficulty is that the best results appear to be obtained using oocytes taken from the largest follicles which are therefore already the most mature in vivo [46] then it may be stored (as an non - licensable activity), in, say, prospective oncology treatment as a form of 'fertility insurance' [47] - (if the HFEA is correct);

- with the consent of the woman if over 18, as with any other adult;
- if 16-18 with consent by the adolescent woman herself; [48]
- with the consent of the adolescent woman herself if she is under 16 and 'Gillick competent'[49] or;
- if not *Gillick* competent then with the consent of her parent(s) or another person with parental responsibility.[50]

It is possible that autografting pieces of ovarian tissue which have been excised and cryopreserved would enable a woman to attempt to conceive without IVF, but if the immature gametes are later taken from the tissue and matured in vitro,[51] then the Act will apply *even if the oocytes are to be used for the woman's own benefit*. Ovarian tissue grafting carries a risk, of course, which is not present with use of frozen mature oocytes, of reintroducing cancerous cells with the transplant.

Merely because the tissue is stored in the course of an unlicensed activity does not mean, however, that it is free from legal control, especially not at the behest of the tissue provider.   Thus where the unlicensed activity takes place - as most will do I suspect - in a clinic outside the NHS, there will be an express or implied contract between the gamete provider and the clinic. The contract might expressly provide what is to happen to the tissue, although the enforceability of a detrimental term against a *minor* would be highly unlikely. More likely might be a claim *against* a clinic for wrongful disposal of the tissue, including a claim that the tissue disposed of belonged - in a proprietary sense - to the provider. Any such (contractual) claim could include a claim for damages for any personal distress caused to the provider by the dealing with the tissue (for example, apparent use or disposal of the tissue without the provider's consent or in breach of the implied terms of the contract).[52]

What would need to be shown to establish a proprietary interest is that there is *'some practical value or possible sensible purpose in retaining the specimen for future use such that it makes sense to recognize a proprietary or possessary interest.*[53] A cryopreserved or otherwise stored immature gamete probably comes as close to illustrating such a consideration as any other tissue is likely to do.

The Human Tissue Act 1961   There is a further issue; concerning the applicability of the Human Tissue Act 1961 to immature oocytes and their use subsequent to the death of the provider. Mature oocytes, or gametes, are of course within the statutory scheme of the HF & E Act.   Gamete donation is within sch 3 para. 2(2) of the Act. But ovarian tissue, on the HFEA's definition of gametes, is not. But it does probably fall within the 1961 Act.[54] The relevant section of that Act is section 1;

> (1) If any person, either in writing at any time or orally in the presence of two or more witnesses during his last illness, has expressed a request that his body *or any specified part of his body* be used after his death for therapeutic purposes ... the person lawfully in possession of his body after his death may, unless he has reason to believe that the request was subsequently withdrawn, authorise the removal from the body of any part, or as the case may be, the specified part, for use in accordance with the request.

> (2) ... the person lawfully in possession of the body of a deceased person may authorise the removal of any part of the body for the said purpose if, having made such reasonable enquiry as may be practicable, he has no reason to believe that,
> (a) the deceased had expressed an objection to his body being dealt with after his death and had not withdrawn it; or

(b) that the surviving spouse or any other relative of the deceased
objects to the body being so dealt with.

S1(1) thus contemplates the direction by a person in their last illness to the
use of a part of their body after death for therapeutic purposes. Where this
concerns the recovery of immature oocytes through follicle puncture or
through ovarian tissue biopsy this may be a way of a person about to
undergo therapy which in the event they do not survive effectively being
able to 'donate' immature oocytes for the use by another woman.[55]

Where a license for storage is needed the effective consents provisions
of the HF & E Act must be complied with. Such consent can only be
provided by the person whose gametes are to be stored; there is no
provision in the Act here for substituted consent. Neither the parents of a
girl unable to provide an effective consent, nor any one else with parental
responsibility can provide an effective consent in such circumstances.

Thus, if it is intended to take ovarian tissue containing gametes *for
storage* as understood by the HFEA the following steps must be complied
with;

it may be stored *only* if there is an effective consent

- by the woman (if over 18); or
- the adolescent woman between 16-18; or
- an adolescent woman under 16 who is *Gillick* competent *herself* to
  give consent to the storage.

The consent of no-one else to the storage will suffice.

With adolescent girls this will mean that in each case the doctor must
be satisfied that the girl is capable of understanding the *implications* of the
proposed course of action. This will mean that:

- the mere written recording of agreement is not sufficient;
- effective consent properly understood will mean that the decision
  has been arrived at on the basis of information and discussion; if
  the clinician concludes that a young woman cannot understand the
  information or is unable to participate in a discussion concerning
  the proposed treatment and the implication of the storage
  (including the possibility that the gametes may later have to be
  allowed to perish) then although he or she might conclude that the
  girl would be *Gillick* competent for a range of *other* therapeutic

interventions, the doctor may yet have to conclude that the young woman is not *Gillick* competent for this proposed intervention;

- that the provisions of Schedule 3 HFE Act have been complied with; thus, that

> A consent under this Schedule must be given in writing and, in this Schedule, "effective consent" means a consent under this Schedule which has not been withdrawn ...

and crucially

> 2(2) A consent to the storage of any gametes ... must
> (a) specify the maximum period of storage (if less than the statutory storage period) and
> (b) state what is to be done with the gametes ... if the person who gave the consent dies or is unable because of incapacity to vary the terms of the consent or to revoke it,
> (c) and may specify conditions subject to which the gametes ... may remain in storage.

It is possible that the risk of *re-introducing* the cancer from the tissue with immature oocytes would need to be raised, if not at the time of taking then at some later time; with frozen oocytes there is, of course, no such risk of transmission.

Whether ovarian tissue contains gametes in any given case will need to be decided by the clinician according to the woman's menstrual cycle or testing of the tissue itself.

This reading of the scope of the Act leads to the conclusion, undesirable as it may be, that there are circumstances in which it would be perfectly lawful to *recover* ovarian tissue containing gametes, or even gametes themselves, at common law (as being in the 'best interests' of someone who was incapable of consenting to their taking), but where it would be unlawful to store them in any way.[56] While this may be a less of a problem in respect of ovarian tissue or oocytes, it is undoubtedly a very great problem in respect of post - Tanner stage 2 boys (infra) who are judged not *Gillick* competent for the purposes of giving effective consent to storage within Schedule 3.

Indeed, it might be thought that this anomaly, as Professor McLean describes it, where gametes might be *lawfully*[57] recovered as being in a person's best interests but may not be stored until such time as they can exercise their own determination as to what they believe their best interests to be might be, provides a clear indication of a provision in a UK statute which is clearly incompatible with the European Convention on Human Rights articles 8 and 12. In relation to any relevant challenge, British courts will soon be required under the Human Rights Act 1998 to pay attention to these provisions.

Indeed, such a restriction on an attempt to preserve gametes prior to the export to another member state for the purpose of longer term storage with a subsequent view to the use of treatment services there, might also be thought to be in contravention of the relevant provisions of Treaty of Rome (as amended). Here, we run into the wider reaching effects of the decision of the Court of Appeal in *Blood*.[58] In deciding that infertility treatment services unequivocally fall within the scope of Articles 59 and 60 (free movement of services),[59] and in doing so in the way in which they did, the Court of Appeal have opened a number of interesting lines of inquiry.

Lord Woolf in the Court of Appeal concluded that in a case where a woman wished to receive artificial insemination using sperm of her late husband,

> ... it is artificial to treat the refusal of permission to export the sperm as not withholding the provision of fertilization treatment in another Member State ...

and concluded that from a functional point of view the ability to provide those services '... is not only substantially impeded but made impossible'. The HFEA's original refusal to permit the export of Mr Blood's sperm '... prevents Mrs Blood having the only treatment which she wants'.[60]

Mutatis mutandi in respect of the storage of gametes or ovarian tissue containing gametes otherwise lawfully recovered which it is said cannot be lawfully preserved. The effect of the consent schedule - otherwise of laudable ambit - produces in the case of someone unable to give effective consent to the storage of that tissue even where it would be *therapeutically* justified - and this is the important limiting condition of this argument - a restriction on them having access to the only treatment which they might [later] want and would infringe as it did in Mrs Blood's case not only the freedom from restriction to *receive* services (itself a right derivative from the freedom to provide services) but also their implied freedom from restriction on the export of *resources necessary to secure those services* (i.e.; in such a case, the cryopreserved or otherwise stored gametes).

Testicular Tissue The HFEA works to the grades of puberty described as the Tanner Grade[61] and advises that the storage of tissue from boys who have reached Tanner Stage 2 or beyond would require a license from the

HFEA and effective consent. Again because substituted consent is not possible under the HF & E Act, consent to storage cannot be given *on* behalf of a child who has reached Tanner stage 2. Thus;

- an adolescent boy of 16 - 18 can give an effective consent to removal and storage of tissue as valid as if he were an adult;
- an adolescent boy under the age of 16 can give effective consent to removal and storage of tissue if he is adjudged by the treating doctor to be *Gillick* competent;

Tissue may be recovered from a boy under the age of 16 who is not *Gillick* competent if it is in his best interests following the consent of;

- a parent
- a person with parental responsibility
- in an emergency if the removal could be deemed to amount to therapy for a boy who is about to undergo treatment which would render him infertile and where he is not expected to recover from that condition.

If a boy is pre pubertal his tissue can be recovered *and stored on unlicensed premises*. In this case the ground for so recovering the tissue is that it will be in the 'best interests' of the minor for it to be recovered. But here it is worth noting the cautious recommendation of the McLean Report;

> ... in the event of doubt as to whether or not the individual will recover, or doubt about whether or not fertility after recovery will be affected, where it is intended to use the 'best interests' test to authorise removal of gametes, clinical staff should be advised that recourse should be had to a court of law for determination of the lawfulness of the proposed removal.[62]

On problems of cryopreservation

It sometimes happens that gametes, or embryos derived from gametes, remain in storage at the death of one or rarely both [63] of the genitors. The surviving party might then nonetheless seek to make use of the stored gametes or embryos. The Warnock Committee wished to see the posthumous use of gametes 'actively discouraged'.[64] The Committee believed that birth in such circumstances might give rise to profound psychological problems for child and mother, and were worried about the lack of finality in the administration of estates which would be engendered by the possibility of such births.[65] It would have been open to the legislature to provide that no such use could be contemplated, but it did not. Instead, the Act provided that if posthumous use of gametes is to be made, the provider has to have given clear *written* indication that that conformed with, and certainly did not go against any specific wishes or views that they held;[66] not surprisingly the mechanism used to ensure this outcome was consent.[67]

One exception to the requirement of formal written consent is where sperm is being used in a treatment service for the benefit of the woman and the sperm provider *together*.[68] Use of gametes in contravention of the consents provisions carries a number of consequences; it may breach the license issued by the HFEA to the 'person responsible' for the clinic where the treatment services are offered, it may amount to a criminal offence and it may affect the status of any child born of those treatment services.[69]

In *Blood*, the Court of Appeal, however, was ready to assist Mrs Blood in her 'agonizing situation'[70] in seeking to make use of sperm which she has caused to be recovered from her dying husband after his death. The legal problem was that Mr Blood appeared to have given no 'effective consent' for the use of his sperm in this way. The Court of Appeal accepted Mrs Blood's argument that the HFEA's decision refusing to make specific directions allowing access to the sperm for export was an interference with her rights under Articles 59 and 60 of the Treaty of Rome.[71] These articles provide that restrictions on one of the Union's four freedoms - here the right to receive services (as a concomitant of the guarantee of freedom of movement) - have at least to be justified by some imperative public interest requirement. Since the HFEA had not given an adequate account of such considerations, they were required to re-consider their decision, taking into consideration principles of EU law and, in the light of the Court's judgment on the legality of preserving sperm without consent, the unlikely possibility of such a case recurring. While stressing the HFEA's dominion of the substantive issue, the Court opined that Mrs Blood's position was 'much stronger' than when the Authority last considered the matter 'the legal position having received further clarification'. Moreover, although not ruling on whether the reasons presently given by the HFEA could pass European scrutiny, Lord Woolf thought this 'unlikely'.[72] So, not only did the Court use the trump of EU law to sweep aside the hand dealt by the UK Parliament, it dealt the cards with which the HFEA must now play, and left the applicant holding all the aces.

These two examples, briefly stated (and they could be added to or multiplied) illustrate the minor thesis here - that the introduction of a statutory regime is far from a panacea for resolving public choice or legal issues in regulating reproduction. They also illustrate one of the necessary complexities which statue introduces; words do not interpret themselves, science does not obligingly stand still and 'patients' demands and expectations are not static. Attempting to paint a picture or take a snap shot of the relationship between law and aspects of medical science may distort what is its essentially fluid, dynamic nature; one which is metaphorically represented better by pentimento than a fixed and unchanging portrait.

VI. General issues down the tube

Nonetheless, I am a great believer that the field of Medical Law as much as Medical Ethics should conform so far as is possible with Bill Bryson's first rule of shopping; you should never buy anything which is too heavy to make the children carry home.[73] In other words, medical law, so far as is possible, should be simple and straightforward and capable of ready understanding in everyday use in the High Street as much as in the High Court. With assisted conception and embryology, the law is coming closer, as I have tried to show, I venture, to Flanders & Swann's view of the second law of thermodynamics than Bryson's more accommodating rule. It is becoming more and more complex and being made to dance upon the heads of embryological spindles.

Medical concern is now inexorably seen as moral concern; medical politics is largely dominated by moral politics,[74] as, indeed, it was from the mid C19 embryonic development of 'medical ethics'; medical welfare was then as now equiparated with moral welfare. While some have argued that health technologies will give rise to new and pressing questions of social regulation and ethics,[75] including social identity and relatedness,[76] others have more sanguinely proposed that developments in reproductive medicine and molecular biology either give rise to no new ethical questions,[77] or that, insofar as they do, the market may provide an appropriate[78] or the only[79] response. One important preliminary question is to delineate the extent to which emergent 'innovative' health technologies could properly correspond to a 'market',[80] quasi-market[81] or 'moral regulation'[82] model, and what, if any significant, difference this might make, either in regulatory terms, or the ends to which such regulation might be directed.[83]

At one level, the clearest *legal* issues are the regulation of the uses of the fruits of scientific knowledge related to addressing infertility. Such fruits might come in at least two palettes;

- changing or modifying existing practices or behavior, whether in relation to individual human patients, their gametes or embryos or gametes or embryos derived from a donor;
- regulation of the circumstances under which embryos derived from these practices may be brought to conception and the information later to be available to those individuals as to the circumstances of their conception.

These are the fairly standard concerns of lawyers who have addressed questions of the regulation of assisted conception. With them come several contributions (usually and necessarily derived from moral philosophy) to understandings of human dignity, 'personhood', and consequential matters relating to the medical or genetic interventions at the beginning of life.

At another level, however, are questions that are predicated upon a different understanding of the role and contribution of law. Here, law is seen not (just) as an autonomous body of knowledge but as a factor which contributes to, which in part translates and facilitates the so called 'public understanding of science' but which also operates in a similar way in contributing to the less well developed enquiry of the 'scientific understanding of the public'.[84] Of course, this may vary according to a number of discrete variables and modes of analysis; is law to be seen as only an instrumental response to assisted conception practices, or is there an ideological, a symbolic element to it as well, or instead?

Here, biomedical diplomacy focuses on the negotiation of the movement from bioethics to biolaw (how and why laws and regulations come to be passed) or from bioethics to biopolitics (how and why some laws and regulations come to be passed and others not). The focus here is on the development and implementation of individual regulatory regimes and the way(s) in which those come to shape negotiation of European (and wider) policies, statements, or rules of international import which seek to address the global availability and impact of defined technologies in the art and practice of medicine. This is an examination of the way in which 'risk societies' seek to comprehend and respond to this manufactured uncertainty.

Work that properly broaches these questions has hardly begun in a serious way; addressing what might be called the sociology of medical law.

To that extent, many of the pertinent questions that we might address in the regulation of assisted conception have hardly been formulated with clarity. Understanding regulating reproduction seriously is a long way down the tube.

Notes

1   Clearly, this draws from and builds on W Felstiner, R Abel and A Sarat, 'The Emergence and Transformation of Disputes: Naming, Blaming and Claiming,' (1980-81) *Law & Society Review,* vol. 15, p. 631.

2   *A People's Tragedy: The Russia Revolution 1891 - 1924* (1996), Pimlico, London, at 733, 857n.

3   Eric Hobsbawm, (1994) *Age of Extremes: The Short Twentieth Century 1914-1991,* Michael Joseph, London, p. 287.

4   This is not to imply that such concerns are exclusive to westernised societies; see, for example, Noel Williams, *The Right to Life in Japan*, (1997), Routledge, London, esp at 5-15 and 85-100; Sir Immanuel Jakobovits, (1986) 'The Jewish Contribution to Medical Ethics' in Peter Byrne (ed), *Rights & Wrongs in Medicine*, King Edward's Hospital Fund for London, London, pp. 115-26, and the papers variously collected in Norio Fujiki and Darryl R J Macer, (1998) *Bioethics in Asia*, Eubios Ethics Institute, Tskuba Science City.

5   A Ogus, (1994) *Regulation: Legal Form and Economic Theory*, Clarendon Press, Oxford; R Baldwin and M Cave, (1999) *Understanding Regulation: Theory, Strategy and Practice*, Oxford University Press, Oxford.

6   See Ogus *op. cit.*, esp chs 3 and 6; F von Hayek, (1973) *Law, Legislation & Liberty*, Routledge & Kegan Paul, London.

7   For an outstanding recent exception see Black 1998, *op. cit.*

8   Morgan and Lee, (1991) *Blackstone's Guide to the Human Fertilisation & Embryology Act 1990,* Blackstone Press, London; Brazier, (1999), *op. cit.*; for an early historical evaluation see Gunning and English, (1993) *Human In Vitro Fertilisation*, Dartmouth, Aldershot; An outstanding exception to the descriptive accounts of the debates is Mulkay, (1997) *The Embryo Research Debate: Science and the Politics of Reproduction*, Cambridge University Press, Cambridge.

9   Morgan and Bernat, (1992)'The Reproductive Waltz: The Austrian Medically Assisted Procreation Act 1992' *Journal of Social Welfare Law*, p. 420; Morgan and Nielsen, (1992) 'Dangerous Liaisons: Law, Technology, Reproduction and European Ethics' in Shaun McVeigh and Sally Wheeler, (eds), *Law, Health and Medical Regulation*, Dartmouth, Aldershot, pp. 52 - 74; Morgan and Nielsen, (1993) 'Prisoners of Progress or Hostages to Fortune?'   *The Journal of Law, Medicine and Ethics*, vol 21 (1), pp. 30-42; Morgan (1998)'Licensing Parenthood and Regulating Reproduction: Towards Consensus?' Cosimo Marco Mazzoni, (ed), *A Legal Framework for Bioethics*, Kluwer Law International, The Hague, at 107 - 118; Nielsen, (1998) 'From Bioethics to Biolaw' in Cosimo Marco Mazzoni, (ed), *A Legal Framework for Bioethics*, Kluwer Law International, The Hague, at 39 – 52; Beyleveld, *op. cit.*

10   Skene, (1999) 'Why legislate on Assisted Reproduction?' in Freckelton and Peterson, eds., *Controversies in Health Law*, The Federation Press, Sydney; Szoke, (1999)

'Regulation of Assisted Reproductive Technology: The State of Play in Australia, in Freckelton and Peterson, eds., *Controversies in Health Law*, The Federation Press, Sydney.

11   Perri (1997), *Holistic Government*, Demos, London.

12   Kock, (1991) IVF - An Irrational Choice?

13   Chalmers, (1999)'The Challenge of Human Genetics' in Freckelton and Peterson, eds., *Controversies in Health Law*, The Federation Press, Sydney.

14   There is a comprehensive examination of various different European regulatory regimes in Deryck Beyleveld and Shaun Pattinson, (2000)'Legal regulation of assisted procreation, genetic diagnosis and gene therapy', in Deryck Beyleveld and Hiller Haker, (eds), *The Ethics of Genetics in Human Procreation*, Ashgate, Aldershot, pp. 215 – 76.

15   After, Health Council of Netherlands Committee on in vitro fertilisation, (1998) *IVF-Related Research*, Rijswijk, at 66.

16   Knoppers and Le Bris (1991) 'Recent Advances in Medically Assisted Conception: Legal, Ethical and Social Issues' *American J of Law & Medicine*, vol. 17., pp. 329-61

17   Albin Eser, (1989) 'Legal Aspects of Bioethics' in *Europe and Bioethics*, Proceedings of the 1st Symposium of the Council of Europe on Bioethics, Strasbourg, , pp.41 at 42. I suspect that I differ from Eser in the extent to which I think this categorisation captures or expresses a dynamic rather than static account of what be called 'the goals of medical law'; but they are for the moment a useful working vocabulary which would need later to be employed in a more mature reflection on the regulation of assisted conception.

18   Following Mme Catherine Lalumiere,(1989) 'Allocutions D'Ouverture' *in Europe and Bioethics*, Proceedings of the 1st Symposium of the Council of Europe on Bioethics, Strasbourg, pp.12-14.

19   See John Griffiths, (1979) 'Is Law Important?', *New York University Law Review*, vol. 54, p. 339.

20   Morgan, (1998)'What does Biomedical Diplomacy Mean? Law, Ethics and the Regulation of Modern Medicine', IV World Congress of Bioethics, Tokyo, Japan.

21   Galanter, (1992) 'Law Abounding' *Modern Law Review*, vol. 55, p.1; Teubner, 1987, 'Juridification: Concepts, Aspects, Limits, Solutions' in Teubner, (ed), *Juridification of Social Spheres*, Walter de Gruyter, Berlin, pp. 3- 48.

22   Guido Calabresi (with Phillip Bobbit), (1978) *Tragic Choices*, W W Norton, New York.

23   Hobsbawm, (1994) *Age of Extremes: The Short Twentieth Century 1914-1991*, Michael Joseph, London, p. 287; Fujiki and Macer, (1998) *Bioethics in Asia*, Eubios Ethics Institute, Tskuba Science City; Kumar, (1987)'Legal Implications of Medical Advancement' in P Leelakrishan and G Sadasivan Nair, (eds.), *New Horizons of Law*, Cochin University of Science and Technology, Cochin, pp.199-212, esp. at pp.199-204 and 210-12; Manga, (1992) 'New Reproductive Technologies in the Third World: Heightened Human Rights and Ethical Controversies' (paper delivered to the *Third International Conference on Health Law and Ethics*, Toronto, July 1992.

24   Wolf, (1994) 'The Rise of the New Pragmatism', *American Journal of Law & Medicine*, vol 20, p. 211; Doyal, (1995) *What Makes Women Sick?*, Rutgers University Press, New Brunswick.

25   Beck, *op. cit.*; Bauman, (1993) *Postmodern Ethics*, Blackwell, Oxford; Bauman, (1995) *A Life in Fragments*, Blackwell, Oxford.

26   *Op cit.*, p. 211.

27   Giddens, (1999)'Risk and Responsibility' *Modern Law Review* vol.61, p. 1.

28   *Ibid* at 3.

29   *Ibid.*

30   de Sousa Santos,(1995) *Toward a New Common Sense*, Routledge, London.

31   Anthony Giddens has recently called this notion 'plastic sexuality'; this is a potentially important analytical dimension in examining assisted conception; see Anthony Giddens, (1992) *The Transformation of Intimacy*, Polity Press, Cambridge.

32   A term coined by Peter Singer and Deane Wells, (1984) *The Reproduction Revolution*, Oxford University Press, Oxford.

33   I have offered an introductory survey to these various approaches in (1998) 'Frameworks of Analysis of Feminism's Accounts of Reproductive Technology' in Sally Sheldon and Michael Thompson, (eds), *Feminist Perspectives on Health Care Law,* , Cavendish Publishing, London), pp. 189-209.

34   Sheila McLean, (1992) 'Reproductive Medicine' in Clare Dyer, (ed.), *Doctors, Patients and the Law*, Blackwell, Oxford, pp.89-105 at p.89.

35   Cook and Dickens, (1998) *Considerations for Formulating Reproductive Health Laws*, World Health Organisation, Geneva.

36   Montgomery (1991) Rights, Restraints and Pragmatism: The Human Fertilisation & Embryology Act 1990, *Modern Law Review*, vol 54, p. 524.

37   H.L. Vol. 516 Col. 1089.

38   Morgan & Lee at p.32.

39   Article 8.2; 'There shall be no interference by a public authority with the exercise of this right except such as in accordance with the law as it is necessary in a democratic society ... for the protection of health and morals, or for the protection of the rights and freedoms of others.'

40   Wadham J and Mountfield H, (1999) *Blackstone's Guide to the Human Rights Act 1998*, Blackstone Press, London at p. 108.

41   *Review of the Common Law provisions Relating to the Removal of Gametes and of the Consent Provisions in the Human Fertilisation and Embryology Act 1990*, Department of Health, London, July 1998.

42   *Surrogacy: Review for Health Ministers of Current Arrangements for Payments and Regulation*, Cm 4068, Department of Health, London, October 1998.

43   London, HFEA & HGAC, 1998.

44   This is a device adopted by other European jurisdictions, for example Denmark and France, in their legislation concerning assisted conception procedures and their regulation. For a recent review of the French legislation of 1994 (Loi 94-654) as required by that Act see   *L'application de la loi no. 94-654 du 29 Juillet 1994*, No. 1407, Assemblée Nationale; No. 232, Sénat; Office Parlementaire d'Evaluation des choix Scientifiques et Technologiquees, 1999.

45   'Storage and Use of Ovarian Tissue' (London, HFEA, 1998). Section 1(4) HFE Act 1990 s1(4) is the closest that the legislation itself comes to a definition; 'references to gametes or eggs do not include eggs in the process of fertilisation.'

46   Health Council of Netherlands, Committee on in vitro fertilisation, *IVF-Related Research*, Rijswijk, 1998, at p. 41, para. 3.2.2.

47   Because s2(2) does not apply by virtue of s1(4); for the notion of 'fertility insurance' see Health Council of Netherlands, Committee on in vitro fertilisation, *IVF-Related Research*, Rijswijk, 1998, at p. 47, para. 3.4.3.

48   Family Law Reform Act 1969 s8 provides;

         '(1) The consent of a minor who has attained the age of sixteen years to any surgical, medical or dental treatment which, in the absence of consent, would constitute a trespass to his person, shall be as effective as it would be if he were of full age; and where a minor has by virtue of this section given an effective consent to any treatment it shall not be necessary to obtain any consent for it from his parent or guardian.'

49   *Gillick v West Norfolk & Wisbech AHA* (1985) *All England Reports*, vol. 3, p. 402.

50   For the concept of 'parental responsibility' see Children Act 1989 s.3.

51   IVM; in vitro maturation of oocytes.

52   *Bliss v South East Thames RHA* (1987) ICR p. 700; *Hayes v Dodd* (1990) *All England Reports* vol. 2, p. 815.

53   *Dobson v North Tyneside Area Health Authority* (1996) All ER, vol.4. p. 464.

54   *Review of the Common Law provisions Relating to the Removal of Gametes and of the Consent Provisions in the Human Fertilisation and Embryology Act 1990*, Department of Health, London, July 1998, p.21, para. 3.13.

55   For present purposes I *assume* that there is no other doubt as to the technical viability of such grafting.

56   And recall that s2(2) of the Act regards cryopreservation as merely one method of storing within the Act. Of course, this is not applicable to immature oocytes, as defined by the HFEA.

57   This limitation is crucial; see *McLean Report* at para. 2.9.

58   *R v Human Fertilisation & Embryology Authority ex parte Blood* (1997) *All England Reports*, vol. 2, p. 687 (Court of Appeal). There is a note of the case by Morgan and Lee in (1997) *Modern Law Review*, vol. 60, pp. 840-56.

59   The jurisprudence of the ECJ on these questions appears quite unequivocal; 'Where rules impede market access by suppliers based in other Member States they must be objectively justified. That the court has not been deterred from developing this principle despite Article 60(3) [permitting the supply of services to be regulated by the host state on 'the same conditions as are imposed by the state on its own nationals'] testifies to its determination to construct a core set of principles of Community trade law, drawing together the separate Treaty provisions, most of all Articles 30 and 59.' Weatherill S, (1995*) Law and Integration in the European Union,* Clarendon Press, Oxford, p. 253.

60   (1997) *All England Reports*, vol. 2, 687 at 700 and 698.

61   'Storage and Use of Testicular Tissue' (London, HFEA, 1998).

62   *Review of the Common Law provisions Relating to the Removal of Gametes and of the Consent Provisions in the Human Fertilisation and Embryology Act 1990*, Department of Health, London, July 1998 at para 1.14.

63   The most publicised example of the death of husband and wife who had had embryos stored is that of the 'Rios' embryos', discussed briefly in John Robertson, *Children of Choice: Freedom and the New Reproductive Technologies.* Princeton University Press, Princetion, NJ 1996 ed., at pp. 111-12, and more extensively in his 'Posthumous Reproduction,' (1994) *Indiana Law Journal* vol. 69, pp.1027-1066, and G P Smith, (1985)'Australian's Frozen "Orphan" Embryos: A Medical, Legal and Ethical Dilemma' *Journal of Family Law*, vol, 24, p.27.9314, para 4.4; it is in light of this that the evidence of (the now) Baroness Warnock comes to be considered. Warnock gave an affidavit, later admitted in evidence, that the Committee had given no consideration to the facts of a case such as that now before the court. In that sense, her affidavit was introduced to seek to persuade the court that Blood was such an unusual set of facts that the Committee had not even been thinking about the desirability or undesirability of what was being proposed at all.

64   *Ibid*, paras, 10.9 and 10.15. For resolution of precisely this point under the Tasmanian Administration and Probate Act 1936 s46(1) see, *In the Matter of the Estate of the*

*Late K and in the Matter of the Administration and Probate Act 1935 ex parte The Public Trustee (*1996) *Tasmania Reports*, vol. 5, p. 365, noted by Morgan D, 'Rights and legal status of embryos' (1996) *Australian Health Law Bulletin*, vol. 4 (7), p.1; Chalmers D, (1996) 'Inheritance Rights of Embryos' *University of Tasmania Law Reports*, vol. 15 (1), p. 131, and Atherton R in (1998) 'Between a Fridge and a Hard Place: The Case of the Frozen Embryos or Children *en ventre sa frigidaire*' *Australian Public Law Journal*, vol. 6 (1), p. 53 and ' Atherton R (1999) '*En ventre sa frigidaire:* Posthumous children in the succession context', *Legal Studies*, vol. 20, p.139.

66   Somewhat cavalierly, Lord Woolf in *Blood's case* at 703 remarks that the legislative provision for written consent '... is not obvious in this situation'.

67   HFE Act 1990, Sch 3, para 1; 'A consent under this Schedule must be given in writing and, in this Schedule, "effective consent" means a consent under this Schedule which has not been withdrawn.'; para 2(2), 'A consent to the storage of any gametes or an embryo must (a) specify the maximum period of storage (if less than the statutory storage period), and (b) state what is to be done with the gametes or embryo if the person who gave the consent dies ... '; para 5(1) 'A person's gametes must not be used for the purposes of treatment services unless there is an effective consent by that person to their being so used and they are used in accordance with the terms of that consent; ... (3) This paragraph does not apply to the use of a person's gametes for the purpose of that person, or that person and another together, receiving treatment services'.

68   HFE Act s4(1)(b). Both the High Court and the Court of Appeal dismissed the argument that although Stephen Blood was dead, he and Diane Blood could nonetheless benefit from the saving in this provision. The HFEA countered that as between Mrs Blood and the stored sperm of Stephen Blood, after his death the sperm fell to be treated as if it were the sperm of a donor, and hence within the licensing regime so as to require the necessary consent. It is arguable (but still not free of doubt) that if it had been the Clinic's intention to provide Mrs Blood with the treatment services as her husband lay dying, immediately before the determination of his death, the marriage would still have subsisted and written consent would not have been required (see, *infra*, p. 39). To the general principles established in English law might now be added the provisions of the Council of Europe, *Convention on Human Rights and Biomedicine (Convention for the Protection of Human Rights and Dignity of the Human Being with regard to the Application of Biology and Medicine)*, Directorate of Legal Affairs, Strasbourg 1997, DIR/JUR (96)14, articles 5 and 6 (1) '... an intervention may only be carried out on a person who does not have the capacity to consent, for his or her *direct* benefit'. (and see E*xplanatory Report to the Convention* ..., Directorate of Legal Affairs, Strasbourg, 1997), DIR/JUR (97) 1, but carrying no explanation of the notion of 'directness'.

69   HFE Act sections 11-14, 17, 18, 41(2)(b) and 27-30 respectively.   The 'status provisions' contained in sections 27-30 are examined in more detail in Morgan and Lee, (1991), *Blackstone's Guide to the Human Fertilisation & Embryology Act 1990: Abortion and Embryo Research: The New Law*, Blackstone Press, London at 152-69; the immediate provision of relevance, s28(6)(b) is discussed there at pp. 156-60 and in Ian Kennedy and Andrew Grubb, (1994) *Medical Law: Text with Materials*, Butterworths, London, 2nd edition, at p. 819.

70   Lord Woolf, in *Blood*, at p. 700.

71   See also *U v W (Attorney General intervening)* (1997) 2 FLR 282.

72   Lord Woolf, in *Blood* at p. 700.

73   Bryson, (1995) *Notes From A Small Island*, Doubleday, London.

74   Hunt, (1999) *Governing Morals: A Social History of Moral Regulation*, Cambridge University Press, Cambridge.

75   Beck, (1992) *Risk Society: Towards a New Modernity*, Sage, London, trans. Mark Ritter; originally published as *Risikogellschaft. Auf dem Weg in eine andere Moderne*, Frankfurt, (1986), p. 204; Hans Jonas, (1974) *Philosophical Essays: From Ancient Creed to Technological Man*, Prentice Hall, Englewood Cliffs; Hans Jonas, (1984) *The Imperative of Responsibility: In Search of an Ethics for the Technological Age*, University of Chicago Press, Chicago; National Science Foundation, 'Biology and Law: Challenges of Adjudicating Competing Claims in a Democracy'.

76   Strathern, et. al., (1993) *Reproducing the Future: Anthropology, Kinship and the New Reproductive Technologies*, Manchester University Press, Manchester; Strathern,(1992) 'The Meaning of Assisted Kinship' in Meg Stacey, ed., *Changing Human Reproduction*, Sage Publications, London, pp.148-69.

77   Clothier, (1992) *Report of the Committee on the Ethics of Gene Therapy*, Cm 1788, HMSO, London.

78   Duxbury, (1996) 'Do Markets Degrade?' *Modern Law Review*, vol.59,p. 331

79   Silver, *Remaking Eden.*

80   Brazier, (1999) 'Regulating the Reproduction Business? *Medical Law Review*, vol. 7, p. 166.

81   Bartlett and Le Grand, (1993) 'The Theory of Quasi-Markets' in Le Grand and Bartlett, eds., *Quasi-Markets and Social Policy*, Macmillan, Basingstoke.

82   Hunt, *op. cit.*

83   Black, (1998) 'Regulation as Facilitation: Negotiating the Genetic Revolution' in Brownsword, Cornish and Llewelyn, *Law and Human Genetics: Regulating a Revolution*, Hart Publishing, Oxford; Propper, (1993) 'Quasi-markets and Regulation' in Le Grand and Bartlett, eds., *Quasi-Markets and Social Policy*, Macmillan, Basingstoke.

84   A useful portmanteau phrase coined by Celia Wells; see her '"I Blame the Parents" Fitting new Genes in Old Criminal Laws', in Brownsword, Cornish and Llewelyn, *Law and Human Genetics: Regulating a Revolution*, Hart Publishing, Oxford, (1998).

18 Regulation of Assisted Conception Services: The Need for Technical Standardization

JENNIFER GUNNING

Assisted reproduction technologies are now widely available throughout Europe and are generally socially accepted as part of the medical services received by the population. In some countries, such as the United Kingdom, France and the Netherlands and, after a delay in implementing legislation, Spain, statutory regulation controls the provision of assisted conception services. In others they are assimilated into public health services with private clinics operating independently alongside. In most, but not all, countries some form of professional self-regulation also exists.

While public demand for the provision of assisted conception services has increased, public opinion on the status of the embryo, at least as expressed by their political representatives and governments, has remained conservative. Evidence for this is shown by the numbers of countries signing the European Convention on Human Rights and Biomedicine and the number of countries having restrictive, rather than permissive, legislation with regard to embryo research. It is as though no link is seen between the two, that is, between clinical provision and research, yet some of the technologies employed in assisted conception are still largely experimental.

The cultural pressures to reproduce are high and lead to a deep psychological and physical need to have children. The advent of IVF was a boon to infertile couples but the arrival of a technological fix for relatively straightforward causes of infertility, such as blocked fallopian tubes, led to a demand for more sophisticated technological fixes to address more complex causes, such as the use of ICSI and its permutations to overcome male factor problems. In countries with a strong research and training base in assisted reproduction technologies infertile couples are probably assured in finding access to treatment of a high technical standard. But demand for such treatment often exceeds supply through the public health services and, in countries such as the United Kingdom, private clinics abound. In the UK all clinics, public and private are regulated and monitored by the Human Fertilisation and Embryology Authority but where similar regulation does not exist clinics outside the public health service may have little supervision. In those countries, without a strong research and training base, public concerns about the status of the embryo are being met through legislation or through the force of the European Convention on Human Rights and Biomedicine but assisted conception services may be available with relatively little monitoring and control. Greece, for example, has ratified the Convention but, as yet, has no regulation either through the state or through professional associations of assisted conception centers. Assisted conception provision has existed in Greece since 1985, when the first IVF center was established, and there are now some 35-40 centers in operation. The only guidelines issued by the Ministry of Health address donor insemination and merely require the use of frozen, quarantined sperm. These guidelines only came into force some four of five years ago following a case of HIV infection following multiple inseminations with fresh sperm. Legislation on assisted conception procedures is now anticipated in Greece but is likely to focus principally on a legal framework for their application and reimbursement.

It is generally agreed that while regulation of assisted conception services is desirable the harmonization of legislation across Europe is not. Different social and cultural attitudes pertain between countries, for instance, as to who should be eligible for treatment and what sort of treatments should be available. For those who can afford it, of course, reproductive tourism can assure access to the highest technical and safety standards but best practice in terms of technical competence, standard of facilities and safety should be assured to all those seeking treatment. As part of the TRAC project a survey was undertaken to investigate the acceptability to those involved in providing assisted conception services of the introduction of some form of European technical and safety standards.

In order to see whether some sort of European harmonization might be achieved on technical and safety standards, a questionnaire was designed and distributed through the Newsletter of the European Society for Human Reproduction and Embryology and also through contact of some of the project partners.

Background Information

The first part of the questionnaire aimed to characterize the respondents. A total of 72 responses was received, distributed across 15 countries, including one from South Africa. The response was strongest from those countries without legislation and with relatively little regulation, Belgium and Italy, and relatively poor from those countries where assisted conception services are already well regulated. Significantly there were no responses from France. Table 18.1 sets out those responses received by country of residence of the respondent.

Table 18.1   Responses received by country of residence of the respondent

Country of Residence	Number of responses
Belgium	17
Czech Republic	1
Denmark	3
Finland	1
Germany	2
Greece	2
Italy	25
Netherlands	4
Norway	1
Portugal	4
South Africa	1
Spain	5
Sweden	1
Switzerland	2
United Kingdom	3

In order to assess awareness of national regulations, respondents were asked whether regulations affecting assisted conception were in force in their country. As might be expected, those respondents living in countries where legislation had been enacted responded in the affirmative. However there was no consensus on whether regulation existed or not from respondents in Belgium, Italy and Portugal. In fact there is no statutory regulation in these countries though professional self-regulation does exist to a greater or lesser extent and ethics committees play a role in controlling the introduction of new technologies. Respondents from these countries varied in their replies from saying that regulation existed, there was no regulation or they did not know. Table 18.2 sets out the total responses to this question.

Table 18.2   Responses as to whether regulation is in force affecting assisted conception

Response	Number
Yes	35
No	32
Do not know	5

The membership of ESHRE is broad and it was hoped that respondents would reflect a variety of occupations associated with assisted conception. This was indeed the case and, although the majority were clinic directors and clinicians, there were responses from a number of other staff associated with clinics. Three responses came from ESHRE members who had no direct association with an assisted conception center. Table 18.3 shows the distribution of respondents by occupation.

Table 18.3   Distribution of respondents by occupation

Occupation	Number	Occupation	Number
ART Clinic director	36	Clinician	9
Embryologist	14	Counselor	1
Nurse	5	Technician	1
Psychologist	2	Clinical geneticist	1
Clinic administrator	1	University researcher	2
Other (not specified)	1		

Information was also sought about whether clinics were operated in the public or the private sector. The majority of respondents came from private sector clinics (42). State funding supported the clinics of 20 respondents and a further 7 replied that their clinics received a combination of state and private funding. Three respondents were not members of clinic staff. Questions were also asked about clinic size. The results giving the distribution of clinic size according to whether the respondent came from the private or the public sector are given below in Table 18.4.

Table 18.4   Clinic size

Size	Private sector clinics	Clinics wholly or partially state funded
More than 1000 Treatments p.a.	7	10
200–1000 treatments p.a.	26	12
Less than 200 treatments p.a.	9	4

Respondents in the public sector tended predominantly to come from large clinics undertaking more than 1000 treatments a year (38.5%) or from medium sized clinics undertaking 200-1000 treatments a year(46.2%). Private sector respondents came primarily from medium sized clinics (62%). Less than 20% of all respondents came from small clinics undertaking less than 200 treatments per year.

Those respondents who were members of clinic staff were asked to give information about consent procedures at their clinic. Most clinics provided written information to patients and asked them to give written consent to treatment but three responses indicated that no written consent was obtained from patients. It was also asked whether independent counseling was available to patients and although independent counseling was offered in the majority of clinics, 11 respondents said that it was not (5 from the public sector and 6 from the private sector) and 5 respondents, including clinicians, did not know (2 public sector, 3 private sector).

All clinics provided standard IVF treatment and all respondents answered that their clinic also provided ICSI. These treatments were accompanied by a variety of other assisted reproduction procedures including GIFT, ZIFT, TESE, TET, embryo cryopreservation, assisted hatching and donor insemination. A surprising number of respondents said that their clinics offered preimplantation genetic diagnosis (13 from the private sector and 10 from the public sector) and 20 indicated that PGD was planned (15 from the private sector and 5 from the public sector).

Research activities

The respondents to the questionnaire were strongly research oriented, 70% of those from the private sector and 73% from the public sector. A wide range of research activities was recorded from both private and public sector respondents. These are set out in Table 18.5 below.

Table 18.5   Research activities in the public and private sectors

Type of research	Public sector	Private sector
Embryos created	2	1
Using spare embryos	8	11
Embryos re-implanted	0	3
PGD	8	11
On immature oocytes at time of collection	8	16
Oocyte maturation	6	13
Oocyte freezing	5	11
Sperm maturation in vitro	0	2
Other sperm factors	1	3
Blastocyst culture	0	2
Psychological research	2	0
Clinical trials	0	2

Respondents from Belgium were the only ones involved in the creation of embryos for research; two from the public sector and one from the private sector. Yet it is interesting to note the volume of research activity in both sectors on immature oocytes, oocyte maturation and oocyte freezing where one would expect that research embryos would need to be created to test the safety of these procedures before interventions on oocytes became general practice. A significant proportion of this work was being undertaken in private clinics in Belgium and Italy.

Technology transfer

The third part of the questionnaire addressed technology transfer and whether there was any control in the way that new technologies were introduced into clinical practice. Respondents were asked whether approval was required prior to introducing new technologies into their clinic and, if so, who from. The majority of respondents from the public sector (81%) indicated that some form of approval was required. In the private sector, however, although the majority indicated that approval was required (57%) a substantial minority (43%) indicated that it was not. Often more than one mechanism of approval was given. By far the most common body from whom approval was sought was an ethics committee. But hospital management and regulatory bodies were also cited. However, there may be some confusion about the term 'regulatory body' since some respondents from Belgium and Italy, which have no legislation and no regulatory body indicated that approval was required from such a body. Where hospital management was involved this was generally in conjunction with an ethics committee. Table 18.6 sets out the responses on approval in the public and private sectors.

Table 18.6   Approval for the transfer of new assisted reproduction technologies

Approval	Public sector	Private sector
Required: Yes	22	24
No	4	18
Not known		1
Mechanism:		
Regulatory body	6	8
Hospital management	6	4
Ethics committee	16	14
Other		

Where 'other' is shown in the table this refers to the private sector only and authorities such as university chancellor, local committee and clinic team were given.

Respondents were also asked how they obtained their skills. In developing their own skills respondents tended to learn from experts in another country or through the literature followed by undertaking their own research or attending workshops. Most respondents developed their skills through more than one of these mechanisms.

Ensuring best clinical practice

Finally, the questionnaire addressed the problem of ensuring best practice across Europe. The large majority of respondents agreed that there would be benefit in having a European training program for practitioners in assisted conception (62) and in having accreditation of professional standards for specific activities such as treatment , laboratory services and counseling (62). Answers to the suggested forms of technical standardization posed in the questionnaire are shown in Table 18.7

Table 18.7   Responses to suggested forms of technical standardization at the European level

Question - Do you think that at European level it would be of benefit to:	Yes	No	Not known
develop an agreed training program for practitioners in assisted conception	62	9	I
have accreditation of professional standards for specific activities in assisted conception units	62	8	2
develop clinic and laboratory protocols for new procedures	60	9	3

A majority also felt that there would be a benefit in developing clinic and laboratory protocols for new procedures though one respondent remarked that rigid protocols may lead to lack of individuality in units; minimum requirements or 'things not to do' might be better.

Respondents were asked who should take the lead if there were to be technical and safety standardization across Europe. The majority of respondent thought that the lead should be taken by professional associations (46) and ESHRE (49); many thought that this should be done jointly. The setting of standards by Health Ministries was only favored by 6 respondents. Other suggestions were the European Commission, national regulatory bodies such as the HFEA and through publications.

Conclusion

The sample covered in the survey was small but was representative of the professions working in the area of assisted conception and of the different legislative and regulatory backgrounds across Europe. One might have expected a high level of resistance to suggestions about European standardization. But, from the views of the respondents to the questionnaire, there appears to be general agreement among those working in assisted reproduction services that there is a need for some mechanism for assuring best practice across Europe. The consensus seems to be that this should be through training and accreditation by professional associations and ESHRE. The logistics of how this might be achieved are not clear and it is unlikely that these bodies would have the resources to undertake such a process. Nonetheless, they are bodies in whom the practitioners who would be monitored would have confidence.

Article 4, on professional standards, of the European Convention on Human Rights and Biomedicine states:

> Any intervention in the health field, including research, must be carried out in accordance with relevant professional obligations and standards.

A role could be played by European professional associations and ESHRE in determining common standards for training and accreditation in assisted conception services. But it might be more appropriate if the European Commission were to find the means to fund and initiative in this area and to support training workshops to ensure that the requirements of article 4 of the Convention are met. This is important given that there seems to be a rapid uptake across Europe of highly technical procedures such as ICSI and PGD.